I0095842

THE LONG HAULER

A BRUTALLY HONEST AND HONESTLY BRUTAL LOOK AT LIVING WITH CHRONIC ILLNESS AND THE HEALING JOURNEY THAT MAINSTREAM HEALTHCARE PROFESSIONALS WON'T TELL YOU.

Copyright @ 2022 Anne Marie Godin

The Long Hauler: A Brutally Honest and Honestly Brutal Look at Living with Chronic Illness and the Healing Journey that Mainstream Healthcare Professionals Won't Tell You

YGTMedia Co. Trade Paperback Edition.
ISBN trade paperback: 978-1-989716-60-1
eBook: 978-1-989716-67-0

All Rights Reserved. No part of this book can be scanned, distributed, or copied without permission. This book or any portion thereof may not be reproduced or used in any manner whatsoever without the express written permission of the publisher at publishing@ygtmedia.co—except for the use of brief quotations in a book review.

The author has made every effort to ensure the accuracy of the information within this book was correct at time of publication. The author does not assume and hereby disclaims any liability to any party for any loss, damage, or disruption caused by errors or omissions, whether such errors or omissions result from accident, negligence, or any other cause. Some names have been changed to protect the identity of persons discussed.

This book is designed to provide information and motivation to our readers. It is sold with the understanding that the publisher is not engaged to render any type of psychological, legal, or any other kind of professional advice. The content is the sole expression and opinion of its author, and not necessarily that of the publisher. No warranties or guarantees are expressed or implied by the publisher's choice to include any of the content in this book. Neither the publisher nor the author shall be liable for any physical, psychological, emotional, financial, or commercial damages, including, but not limited to, special, incidental, consequential or other damages. Our views and rights are the same: You are responsible for your own choices, actions, and results.

Published in Canada, for Global Distribution by YGTMedia Co.

www.ygtmedia.co/publishing

To order additional copies of this book: publishing@ygtmedia.co

Developmental editing by Kelly Lamb
Edited by Christine Stock
Book design by Doris Chung
Cover design by Michelle Fairbanks
ePub edition by Ellie Silpa

TORONTO

THE LONG HAULER

A BRUTALLY HONEST AND HONESTLY BRUTAL LOOK AT LIVING WITH CHRONIC ILLNESS AND THE HEALING JOURNEY THAT MAINSTREAM HEALTHCARE PROFESSIONALS WON'T TELL YOU.

ANNE MARIE GODIN

Dedicated to:

This is how it always is: You open a book and the dedication is not for you. Not this time.

All those individuals who are the warriors, the long haulers fighting the fight, this is for you. I'm pulling back the cloak of invisibility. I see you.

Jeffery, who has always shown never-ending love, support, and patience for everything I aspire to be or do.

Jason, Joshua, and Jordan, who inspired me as a mother and human to be the best I can be with open eyes and full heart.

Nash, my joy, whom solidified my belief that my story is not over.

The beautiful, intelligent daughters who have merged into my journey along the way.

Ellen DeGeneres, who was always capable of making me laugh when life didn't seem laughable.

TABLE OF CONTENTS

There are many more chapters to unfold in life and much more unconditional love to embrace and joy to behold.

No, this can't be happening! It's so surreal—it's as if I'm reliving a continual loop in a nightmare. I read the article again to digest it all. My eyes are swimming in tears as the words blur together. The lump in my throat is so tight that I can barely take a breath. I weep for those yet to realize their fate. I weep for those living this moment in time. I weep for myself, a long hauler, many years before COVID-19 ever touched humanity.

INTRO

The term "long hauler" has been used extensively to refer to those living with the aftereffects of COVID-19, but it really applies to anyone who has been living with chronic disease. Because when you have chronic illness, you're in it for the long haul! This book is meant to shine light on the invisible and make them more visible for all to see and feel. I welcome you into the healing journey that mainstream healthcare professionals won't tell you about.

Life is not linear, and neither is the path from chronic illness to healing. Why? It's complicated. Chronic illness doesn't just impact the physical and mental well-being of the person who is ill, it affects, in various degrees, all the people they have relationships with. There isn't a singular area of a chronically ill person's life that doesn't get touched, sometimes mangled, by disease. Sometimes parts of their life just disappear. It can be a long, lonely, difficult, and frustrating road, and bringing the journey of healing to others has felt like my destiny. I felt more than ever that this was the moment in time to share my story. After everything I've been through and everything I've learned along the way, I have so much to bring to the table. To do so, I had to take a giant leap in growth to release this manuscript I held so close to my heart.

In the past, I had always viewed vulnerability from the painful side of life because it was often used against me. This internal battle to reconcile vulnerability with strength, however, is so much bigger than just me. To fight the best fight, you have to remove the weakest link. Tossing the link—my vulnerability—out the damn window was the best choice, the only choice, in helping me on my journey. In truth, this pivot has made my vulnerability a strength to bring focus, clarity, and connection to the chronically ill. You're not alone. I hear you. I see you. I am sharing the good, the bad, and the raw ugliness that caused wounds in many areas of my life that made me feel like I would never make it, let alone heal.

More than a decade ago, an invisible disease swept into my life, unexpectedly and unannounced, and it unleashed havoc. In a matter of days, my life as I knew it was utterly upended. It was really scary. The invisibility of it and the threat of death was terrifying. They brought out the paddles on more than one occasion.

It was endless, unpredictable, and unrelenting. The longer this invisible disease continued, the deeper its damaging tentacles grabbed hold of my life. I lost my career, my financial stability. I lost my freedom and my connection to friends, and some friendships and family relationships were irretrievably broken. I lost my ability to eat what I wanted. I was housebound for almost a year and a half. I was filled with anxiety. Would we be able to pay our bills? What was my future going to look like? Was I going to survive this? Was my family going to survive this, both emotionally and financially? Would I live or would I die? None of this was okay. None of this felt right. I just wanted my life back to normal. I wanted me back. I finally have a new normal, but since COVID-19, I've had to adjust my new normal to flow with the current normal. The pandemic required a new pivot.

Does any of what I'm saying resonate with you?

I am here to tell you a few things. Number one, you are going to be okay! Right now, it might not feel that way. But things are going to be alright. Number two, stop being so hard on yourself. Things right now are difficult, and you deserve to give yourself a pat on the back and recognize you are doing the best you can—and that is good enough. Number three, do your best to stop living in your past. This is where you are now, and the quicker you start to focus on the present rather than the past or the future, the better off you will be. You cannot control the events of the situation. The best you can do is risk management and try to control how you react day to day. Last, but not least, number four, you are reading these words, which means you are alive.

Please take time to recognize that you need several things to survive: oxygen, food, water, shelter. So, let's break that down to just one thing—you need your health. That is the one thing that should be your priority. I will not lie. When this pandemic is all done, there will be a new normal. One that you should try not to judge or compare to your old normal or the normal of others around you. When this is done, you should try to remember that most of humanity will adjust, but some will not.

You have the choice to make your life after chronic illness, after COVID-19, the best it can be. It starts with your state of mind. Gratitude, positivity, and hope can go a long way. Right now, you will just have to take my word for that. Hopefully, my story will help in some way.

Buckle up: the journey is going to be a bumpy, eye-opening, profound, and life-changing one.

Sincerely,

Anne Marie, a.k.a. The Long Hauler

PREFACE

FALL 2021

It's September. The air is cool, and the leaves have already started to give way; their vibrant greens fade to shades of yellow and orange. Normally, I love fall—the hues of maple trees cresting on the horizon, finishing their season in a blaze of glory.

I look out over the water and watch the loons float gently as they bob up and down with ease on the waves of our lake. "Ah, to be a loon and just go with the flow."

My Yorkies, Ruby and Alfie, are snuggled up close without a care in the world. Their tiny damp noses are pressed against my thigh to detect any slight movement.

If you would have told me fifteen years ago that this is where I would be, I would have shaken my head and laughed at your premonition. My life, my career, my goals were all mapped out. But it all changed in the blink of an eye, and here I am in this moment in time. My words became writing. My writing became a manuscript.

My cathartic journey needs to find its true destination in the hands of others to read. For so long, I held it tight, not wanting to let it go. To share brings all those tiny flaws and cracks to the surface. To share makes me vulnerable.

To share opens a window for others to see the depth of my journey.

THE DEPTH OF MY LOSSES.

MY SORROWS.

MY HEARTACHE.

MY STRUGGLE.

MY DISEASES.

IT ALSO BRINGS ME FULL CIRCLE TO THE DEPTH OF MY GRATITUDE.

MY STRENGTH.

MY LOVE.

MY TENACITY AND COURAGE TO PIVOT.

Dear Reader, to you I say, life is a journey, and everyone's is different.

Even if we all seem to be on the same page in connection, the level of perception is based on how you have handled the journey thus far and your realization that this moment in time is just that: a moment in time that will pass and lead to the next steps in your journey.

What I learned, trust me, I fought.

One must surrender to things that are out of their control.

When I typed those words, my logical brain said, "Damn, logic tells you to just surrender."

My heart, however, trudged and mourned and trudged some more. I wish I hadn't wasted so much of my time and focus on what I had lost and could not control and instead focused more on taking steps and finding gratitude for what I could control.

I had zero intention of writing a book. Yet there I was from the very beginning of my huge bump in my journey. To be honest, it wasn't a bump, it was more like I had unknowingly taken a wrong turn on a dark curvy bend and drove over a cliff. Flailing arms reaching, trying to grip tightly as everything slipped away. So, I wrote and wrote like my life depended on it. In hindsight, maybe it did. It was cathartic.

I wrote as if someone was reading it, taking it in, listening to me. Digesting my words and sharing:

MY PAIN.

MY STRUGGLES.

MY DISEASES.

Being the optimistic, logical, type A personality doesn't lean well into illness/disease. This is me—go, go, go! Got to do it all. Need to push myself to be the best I can be. Goals are made to be accomplished. I'm a high achiever and never throw in the towel. Yet there I was bedridden, feeling broken, battered, and struggling in so many ways. My body had betrayed me. After the realization that I survived, I was motivated to write. My mind was trying to make sense of it all, my thoughts leaning into "there must be a reason for all this." Whatever the reason, my logical brain needed to find a reasoning as to:

WHY ME?

WHY NOW?

WHY IS THIS HAPPENING TO ME?

WHY? I PLAYED BY ALL THE RULES.

WHY? WHAT DID I DO TO CAUSE THIS?

WHY ME?

SOMEONE? ANYONE? PLEASE TELL ME, WHY?

In hindsight, I can see that getting stuck in the "why" of it all was destructive to my being, to my core, to my relationships. All the unanswered questions. The unexamined narratives that run through your mind that trigger a whirlwind tornado of emotions that wreaks havoc on anything that gets in the way, yourself included.

One can lose themselves in the "why me?" But once I realized that there are unimaginable numbers of individuals who have had their life turned upside down by illness/disease, I changed the question to "why not me?" After all, I'm human, and illness and disease aren't always selective. They don't care who you are.

Changing the narrative moved me in the direction of thinking, *this is where I am; accept it and pivot.* But doing so opened Pandora's box. The one we all keep. The one with bits of baggage all tucked away, compressed like a jack-in-the-box until one too many cranks of the handle and all hell breaks loose. Everyone has baggage or triggers and has used various coping skills or vices to render them into submission. When you suddenly become ill, all your other troubles and heartache don't just go away. They emerge as the unresolved parts of your life, parts of what made you who you are. In my case, it became very clear, very fast, that my vice was food. I didn't have wonderful coping skills; I used food to numb every emotion known to me. It was a learned coping mechanism, one I'm not alone in.

But as my illness gained momentum, so did my emotions: past, present, and future. I called it the balancing scales of life. On one side is the joy, happiness, love, peace, and gratitude; on the other is sadness, depression, pain, grief, hopelessness, anxiety, and disease. In short, we can just call it the shit side of the scales.

My balancing scales were heavily weighted on the shit side of life. I've had struggles throughout my life, yet I coped and didn't miss a beat. Now, it was a whole new ball game. Being abruptly tossed off balance, I soon realized that if one doesn't have their health, nothing else matters. Furthermore, there seemed to be little I could do about that, which made me feel hopeless. My coping mechanisms were nonexistent.

I had a deeply profound awakening once I realized that food was my drug of choice. I had used food my entire life as my number one go-to for coping. Food allergic response came part and parcel with my disease, meaning that I couldn't eat. But for me, food equaled coping—so I couldn't cope. I felt like I had so much work to do. As I peeled back one layer at a time of my emotional onion, another appeared, unresolved and wanting ice cream, bread, pasta, and wine.

I also had the realization that I needed to get in touch with my emotions. To learn, really, what emotion I was feeling and acknowledge that my anger was not the first emotion I was feeling. Often, before we get to the emotion of anger, there is an emotion that happens prior, be it sorrow, fear, shame, sadness, or grief.

We are all complex individuals, whether we like to admit it

or not. I am usually linear in thought. I had planned out my life and goals, and everything went somewhat in the direction I had intended—until it suddenly and abruptly didn't.

One of the deepest and most difficult things to grieve is losing oneself. The loss is profound, heart wrenching, and life altering. Grieving that loss is a process that can feel like it's filled with minefields. Yet when you reach the point of pivoting, know that you have turned toward one of the greatest directions of growth.

As you read through this book, I ask you to keep an open mind. Embrace growth in the manner in which it presents itself. If you have chronic disease, try to accept who and where you are in this moment, and allow yourself to pivot. Give yourself the permission to pivot. Try not to cling to all the expectations of who you thought you were. Trust me, you are so much more than your expectations could ever imagine.

YOU ARE DEEPER.

STRONGER.

MORE COURAGEOUS.

AUTHENTIC.

The universe has said pivot. You can either fight what you cannot control or embrace the pivot to find out you are so much more than you thought you were.

Above all, kindness starts with you. Be kind to yourself.

CHAPTER 1

ACT I—MY LINEAR LIFE

Life is linear, is it not? Nope! What a wake-up call. I have no idea where or why I came up with that concept. I'm sure my therapist and countless others would love to chime in on that one.

In short, I constructed my life in a linear fashion. I made a direct path toward my goals and thought this would mean that I'd avoid all the minefields of life. It seemed like a great concept and gave me easy rules to play by to succeed.

Little did I know that a) life doesn't work that way, and b) we don't all play by the same rules.

My linear mind was constructed from the early stages of life, from newborn to late teens. No one said, "Think linear and you will not only survive but also thrive." I won't get into my childhood or teens—that could be a whole other manuscript.

What I will say is that I am not an individual who hasn't been without troubles or trauma throughout life from childhood right into my twenties. But trauma is a spectrum. Simply put, if something was deeply distressing or disturbing to an individual, then it is trauma. And I had trauma, as many others have, but I don't consider myself a victim, and therefore, I do not adhere to the victim mentality. A warrior? Yes! A survivor? Yes!

My drive and warrior attitude has served me well throughout life. My linear mind has helped me set goals and accomplish more than I could have imagined.

I never used to think about the importance of pivoting in life because there was never any need to when things moved forward the way they were meant to in my linear life, in my linear mind. It's only now, as someone living with chronic illness, that I see how every heartbreak along the way has made me stronger and required me to pivot to endure, to continue. Reflecting on my life has made me realize how often I had to pivot, to adapt, to change so I could continue. And every pivot helped make me stronger, so when I was faced with unbearable difficulties and heartbreak, I was able to go on. I was able to live.

I'm going to share my story so you can see that you're not

alone in your despair. You're not alone in needing to dig deep at times so you can move forward when you don't think you can. We all have stories that shape us and inform how we deal with each difficulty that comes our way on the twists and turns of our not-so-linear lives.

I fell in love with my childhood sweetheart. I mapped out our life together as any love-struck teen would: finish education, get married, buy a house, then have children. When I think about that right now, I realize that I learned to pivot right from the get-go. Not only that, my life didn't go in a linear order. But it all turned out the way the universe wanted it to, and hell yes, thank the stars it did.

Was there pain along the way? Yes! Heartache? Yes!

Life was plugging along. We were married, we had two wonderful boys, and we were taking the steps to buy a brand-new townhouse. Money was tight, but we were happy. We had a busy household with dogs and with me doing carpool in my "mom van."

I loved everything about motherhood. I didn't even mind the diapers and night nursing. I was what I would call a "try and do it all mom." I sewed curtains, made Halloween costumes, baked cookies, planned life and every celebration around wonderful meals for which I made menus and decorated for each occasion. I relished at getting my hands on the latest issue of *Martha Stewart Living*.

We had a warm, tightly knit family life, one I crafted and worked very hard at. The boys brought great joy into my life. Joy had always been scarce and short-lived previously. As they started to grow from infants to little boys, my heart ached horribly to have a little girl. I wanted to share, bond, and empower a daughter. And a daughter was what I'd planned next for my linear life.

Science had made wonderful progress in infertility, and it was possible to actually increase the odds of gender determination. I knew it was a subject that ruffled some feathers, but the fact was, I didn't (and don't) care. My heart wanted what I felt I needed in my life, and damn it all if I wasn't going to give it the best shot at making it happen. I set up the appointment. I was more than eager to put the steps in place so I could have a little girl. The shots were painful, and the endless ultrasounds time consuming. Planning had to be precise, and my poor husband was put on call to produce, which he did. Then his sperm was washed and divided into X and Y.

Like magic, I was pregnant. But this pregnancy was different right from the start compared to my earlier ones with both boys. Every smell made me wretch, but I was elated. We were moving into a brand-new house, and everything was going along pretty smoothly—until it wasn't.

I started spotting at twelve weeks. I was rushed in for an ultrasound. I held my breath as the technician smeared gel over my slight baby bump, and I waited until the monitor beeped the heartbeat. Silent tears of relief eased their way out of the corners of my eyes.

The technician said, “Ah, you are having twins.”

I was shocked, excited, and terrified all at the same time. I giggled at the thought of having twin girls. Double trouble. I took the ultrasound printout and made my way up to the specialist’s office to wait for the overall results.

The doctor looked up at me, barely making eye contact. “The spotting should stop. Just rest.” He quickly waved me out the door.

I woke a few weeks later to cramping and more than spotting. I was sixteen weeks along and gripped with fear. I was rushed in for an emergency ultrasound.

Again, I held my breath until the monitor beeped in rhythm with the babies’ heartbeats. I glanced at the monitor and tried to make out the grainy image. The technician patted my arm and asked me to head back up to the specialist’s office.

I quickly made my way up the flight of stairs with my mind racing and overanalyzing this moment in time. I asked myself why the tech didn’t give me the ultrasound picture printout. I sat impatiently waiting for my turn with a roomful of pregnant women. They all looked further along than I was; some seemed ready to give birth any day. My mind continued to race as I fought back the tears. I barely registered when the nurse called out my name.

Methodically, she motioned and said in a monotone voice, "Room two, gown on, nothing from the waist down. The doctor will be with you shortly."

The doctor knocked, entered with a smile, and patted me on the arm. I thought to myself, *two pats on the arm within an hour. It can't be good news*. The doctor gave me a quick check over and pulled back the curtain so I could dress. I sat in the retro chair, its black vinyl sticking to my sweaty legs. My hands gripped the seat as I waited for the doctor to make eye contact with me.

"Well, I see that you are having girls. The gender has been notated by the technician. I am sorry to say that you have miscarried one, but the other is still viable. It's called 'vanishing twin syndrome' and is quite common in the first and second trimesters." His eyes never left the screen as he quickly said, "I will see you in a few weeks. Get bed rest, and let's see how things go over the next few weeks."

With that, I was dismissed. I sat there trying to process all his words.

TWINS.

GIRLS.

MISCARRIAGE.

VIABLE.

VANISHED.

BED REST.

I didn't want to move. I walked carefully to the car. I chose not to wear my seatbelt, thinking that any undue pressure might be too much. My heart ached. I slowly drove the fifteen minutes home as tears streamed down my cheeks. Bed rest. How does one do that with two active little boys and a house to pack for an upcoming move?

I did my best for the next few weeks, packing only small items. I moved gingerly from the bed to the sofa. Feet up, not lifting anything. The spotting had stopped. I had lost one twin already, the vanishing twin. She just vanished, absorbed back into me and her growing sister. There was no known reason for the loss. With my focus on the future, I cradled my belly and followed the doctor's orders.

The baby was moving, and I was again elated. We were all packed up and ready to move into our newly built home in Courtice, Ontario, a city east of Toronto. It was tranquil in 1990, with farm fields everywhere. It had a real "small town" feel to it. I was overjoyed with the thought of taking the children to pumpkin patches and county fairs.

My pregnancy was moving along, and once I hit week twenty-nine, I no longer felt sick in the mornings. And I didn't feel overly tired. One day, I sat watching the boys playing with matchbox cars around the mountains of boxes filled with all our worldly possessions. I sipped my hot tea and lowered the warm mug to the right side of my belly. She usually moved over instinctively to the warmth. I waited. Then I waited some more. I put down the mug, trying not to worry.

"I'm overreacting," I said to myself.

I rubbed my hands quickly to generate heat and placed them on either side of my rounded belly. I waited. Nothing! Trying not to panic, I called the specialist's office.

His receptionist abruptly announced, "The doctor isn't available; he's in delivery. Give your family doctor a call."

I quickly dialed her number and was ever so relieved when her receptionist picked up the phone and indicated that she would speak with my doctor and get back to me. As I readied the boys to be dropped off at their grandma's, the phone rang. My family doctor had requested I go straight to the hospital; she had arranged for an ultrasound. She was on call and would be available after lunch.

I made my way to the ultrasound department, plopped myself gently between two pregnant women, and eyed a man in a gown as he held his belly in pain. I waited alone in the sterile halls, noticing every smell and nick in the once pristine terrazzo flooring.

When my name was called, I gowned up. I knew the routine all too well: nothing on from the waist down, gown opening in the front.

I stood there, looking down at my naked self. Gently, I touched my belly, stroking it as if touching her beautiful little face, cherub cheeks, pouted lips, and stunning blue eyes. I rendered her vision in my head.

Softly I whispered, "Please don't do this to Mommy. Please don't scare me so."

The cubicle door slammed slightly next to mine. My eyes brimmed with tears as I focused on the door. My thoughts made no sense at all as I noticed how the cubicle was exactly the same as a washroom cubicle minus the toilet.

I stared at the little chrome latch, not wanting to turn it. Not wanting to take a step further. I raised my eyes to the florescent lighting and did something I never liked to do: "God, this is me, Anne Marie. I know I don't talk much to you, and I rarely ask anything of you. But . . . today, I am asking you . . . begging you, please make sure our baby girl is healthy and growing. Please. I will never ask for anything again. Please. I beg you."

"We're ready for you, Mrs. Kewell."

My mind jolted back to reality. The gel felt cold and thick as the tech waved her wand over and over. I held my breath and waited for the monitor to beep in rhythm to my baby's heartbeat.

"How far along are you, Mrs. Kewell?" the tech asked.

"Twenty-nine weeks." I paused. "Where is the heartbeat? Why isn't the monitor beeping? I started off with twins. I already lost one, isn't that enough heartache?" The tears rolled down my cheeks as I continued rambling and questioning the ultrasound tech.

She inhaled sharply, put down her wand, and patted my arm.

"Your family doctor is here. Can you just wait here for a

moment?" Her face couldn't hide the words I feared hearing.

My doctor emerged within minutes. She smiled softly at me and said, "Let's have a look together and go over all the results."

She turned the machine back on and waved the wand over my beautiful, fully rounded belly and pointed to the screen.

The silence of no heartbeat was broken by the click of the machine being turned off. I saw the doctor's lips move.

"I'm sorry, you have lost the baby."

I was in shock. I couldn't believe it. My protest started off as a whimper. "Check it again. The tech is wrong." Then I became more demanding. "Check it again! She's wrong. I have no blood, no spotting. She's wrong! You're all wrong!"

The doctor flipped on the machine and turned the screen toward me. She pointed to my little bundle, resting peacefully. No movement. No heartbeat.

Their words of condolences were drowned out by the depth of my wails, echoing off the sterile walls that closed into darkness.

Somewhat still foggy from being sedated, I drove home four hours later, alone in my minivan with the infant seat clashing around in the back. The seat wasn't packed for the move. Instead, it was waiting for the installation to bring our beautiful daughter home in a few weeks.

The next days were a wash of emotions. I was inconsolable. Going from bed to sofa, back to bed. They made me wait and carry her for two full days before they could assist with her entrance and exit from this world. My husband tried his best to keep the boys distracted and their questions at bay.

The day came. I dropped off the boys and made my way to the hospital, alone. My husband worked, and we couldn't afford for him to take time off. Sometimes you just dig in and do what needs to be done. Sometimes doing it alone takes more out of you than you ever imagined.

The blur of it all. I was all out of tears. I lay dehydrated, staring at the huge light that had been strung overhead. I was calm. I was numb. Void of all emotion, I barely moved when a tray was knocked over and hit the floor. The nurse looked at me sadly.

"You're going to be all right, honey. Do you have any children at home?"

In that moment, panic set in, waves of anxiety rolled over me.

"I didn't tell the boys I loved them before I left!" My voice sounded high-pitched and panicked. The voice didn't sound like my own. The strong me. The confident me. The voice sounded like a stranger, unfamiliar, filled with fear, weak, and vulnerable, sharing openly for all in the room to hear.

The heart monitor beeped quicker and quicker. All medical staff focused their direction on it as the doctor walked in.

"Holy shit, is that her heart rate? Put her out. Now!"

I awoke to the same beeping heart monitor, but now it was a slower rhythm. The nurse took my vitals and said I would be ready to go home in an hour.

Groggy, I glanced up at the nurse and asked to hold my baby girl. I needed to say, "Hello, goodbye, and Mommy loves you more than you will ever know." I wanted to hold her little hand with my pinky finger and kiss her forehead. I wanted to see her beauty and imprint it in my mind, tattooing it on my heart forever.

"Oh, honey, the baby's gone. They took her away hours ago. You don't need to put yourself through that. There will be more. You are young. The baby is with God now," she said and smiled softly.

"There is no God," I announced as I turned my head away from her. The tears didn't fall, but the anger did rise, as it fit too easily into the hole in my heart.

The day passed in pain that etched in my mind. The weeks after were a blur. At my six-week checkup with the specialist, I sat motionless and tearless in the waiting room. My silent lips were tight as I sat in a room full of pregnant women and waited my turn. I glanced down at my flat belly, instinctively touching it softly as if the baby were still there. I knew in my mind that there was no baby. My heart, however, was broken and ached as if the shattered pieces would never be whole again.

The other pregnant women made their way one at a time.

"Room 1, Room 2, Room 3. Mrs. Kewell, the doctor will see you in his office," his nurse announced. The other soon-to-be mothers stared at me as I made my way to the end of the hall.

I sat silently waiting for the doctor to ramble on, hearing very little of what he said other than snippets of the words that rolled off his tongue.

"Twenty-nine weeks, twins. Girl lost at sixteen weeks; girl lost at twenty-nine weeks," he said, his eyes never leaving the computer screen.

"Why? I need to know why?" My voice trembled as I held back the tears. I glared at the doctor as if it were his fault. My anger was reaching its boiling point.

"You had pneumonia. That's why you were prescribed antibiotics. That's why they did a scan when you were in the hospital after you lost the first baby. That's why you had broken ribs. You were coughing so hard you broke ribs," he said, staring at me.

My mind raced, my thoughts were jumbled. I tried to put all his words into order so my brain could make sense of his response.

"So, what the hell does that have to do with me losing the baby?"

The doctor shifted uncomfortably a few times in his seat as he paused to choose his words. Leaning toward me, his lips parted, then closed. It was the first and last time he made eye contact.

"Mrs. Kewell, you coughed so hard you broke ribs. It also pulled the placenta away from the uterine wall. The baby was cut off from oxygen and nutrients." His tone didn't change.

Time stood still. Life stood still. I was numb. The numbness grew like a black weighted cloud that hung over me, suffocating every ounce of my being.

NOTE TO SELF

Speak, even if your voice trembles!

People need to stop giving advice to parents on how to handle the loss of their child. Don't diminish the loss by indicating there will be more. Parents haven't lost an object that can just be replaced. It is a child that has died. Acknowledge the loss of a child, their child, their loss. Stand with them through the grieving process. Be kind, show empathy and compassion, and validate their feeling of the loss of their child. Hold space for them.

TAKE A MOMENT FOR YOURSELF

Breathe, Pause, Reflect . . .

(I have saved a little space for you to make notes if you wish.)

Are you an over-planner?

Did you think your life would be relatively linear?

Think back. When was the first time you recall making a pivot in life?

What feelings did it evoke?

When was the last time you lived in the moment without any expectations?

If you have not lived in the moment (a full day or two) without any expectations, maybe you should give it a try.

Have you ever suffered grief so deeply that you never thought you would recover?

When you think about the loss, are your thoughts from the wound or from the scar?

Glennon Doyle writes that when the wound is open and raw, you can be easily triggered. The healing hasn't fully been accomplished. When the wound turns to a scar, you still know the pain is there, but you can reflect on it with different eyes. You can reflect and still feel the hurt, but when you feel the scar, it doesn't disrupt your life and relationships because it's healed. You have healed. The transition from wound to scar is a major pivot, and one that I would make again and again throughout my life.

CHAPTER 2

THE BURBS FOR A FAMILY OF FIVE

We moved into our new three-bedroom home. I closed the door that would have been the nursery. The boxes marked "Jenna" sat in the garage unpacked, untouched. Weeks turned into months as we finally got organized in the new home. My heart was still broken. My "happy face" mask was on, and I was pretending that all was okay.

I had heard enough people voice their thoughts about how we should try for a girl after having two boys. I always bit my tongue. I suddenly and unexpectedly found myself pregnant again six months later. I didn't tell anyone. I didn't want to get excited. Almost every woman on our block was pregnant, five of us all living next door to one another. The joke was that it must be in the water. I was showing, yet my heart still held back. My heart couldn't take any more breaking than it had already endured.

The boys and Jeff were sick with colds. I was the only one healthy in the household. Prescriptions were ordered for them. Jeff was asleep in bed, so I took the boys with me to pick up all their prescriptions. We waited in line at the pharmacist's counter. People in front, people in back. The boys wouldn't stand still, and I was always reaching for one or the other to keep them in eyesight.

A well-dressed woman in heels giggled as she watched me struggling to keep the boys in line, wiping their noses and telling them to cover their mouths when they coughed. I couldn't wait to get out of there. The cost of the prescriptions gave validation that one of us needed medical coverage. I held my breath, as I feared the amount would cause a decline on my bank card. It didn't, much to my relief. I turned to leave, and the same woman was seated behind us. She tapped her foot on the floor with her stilettos, crossing her legs in one fluid moment.

She glanced up at me and made a clicking with her tongue as if to get everyone's attention. She smirked in a sarcastic kind of way. "Looks like you have another bun in the oven. Bet you have your hopes up to finally have a girl so you can call it quits, eh?" She pointed at my baby bump.

I just stared at her. From somewhere inside, a strong controlled voice projected a response.

"Not that it is any of your business, but I am not waiting to have a girl. I already had my girl. Her name was Jenna. She passed away." I stared her and anyone else who dared to look my way as I exited the store.

Jenna was no longer just some baby who had passed. I gave her an identity, one that she deserved. I owned the pain. I grieved. I surrendered to the thought of "this is where I am right now." I allowed myself to not get caught up in the why of it all.

I quickly, too quickly, moved on with life. One by one, each neighbor gave birth. Four out of five had been born. All girls. I was the last to give birth on a freezing February day. My pregnancy had been up and down. Spotting, bleeding, bed rest, and early labor, a repeat of the last pregnancy to the T with one wonderfully amazing exception. I had a three-hour hard labor and delivered the most beautiful baby boy with the bluest of eyes, as big as quarters. My rainbow baby. My heart burst with joy.

But joy is sometimes fleeting, and I sunk into the "baby blues," as they call it. Months had passed. In hindsight, my husband and I can now say it was postpartum depression that lasted for well over a year. In 1992, it wasn't something that was talked about. Honestly, we didn't even know there was such a thing.

If therapy was available specifically for postpartum, then we didn't know about it, nor would we have been able to afford it. The postpartum depression hung over me like a suffocating wet blanket. I walked the halls at night, as I couldn't sleep. When I could sleep, I had spent hours earlier crying into my pillow, trying not to wake my husband. Deep sobs that made my body shake. My chest was sore from trying to hold it all in. Crying into the damp pillow brought on my asthma. Trying to stifle the asthma cough, I would walk from the upstairs bedroom to the main level of the house, then to the basement, so I could ugly cry into and alternately punch a pillow.

Just to be clear, I adore my boys. They are the light of my life. They have always been my joy and still are to this day. Knowing this, the narrative in my head was one of guilt. I had zero excuse to be that unhappy. The narrative ran in a loop. I had three healthy, wonderful boys, and a great guy of a husband. I lived in a nice home, in a nice neighborhood, in a great country. I had zero reason to be that horrifically, hopelessly unhappy. Yet I was.

We kept thinking it would pass. Our marriage was very rocky. I wanted to leave, thinking that separation would make me happier. I also wanted more children. Truthfully, I still held onto my longing to have a girl. I wanted it even more then. The older boys were bonding with Jeff, and everything was about hockey. I felt constantly bombarded by images of little girls, and by friends who had daughters. My heart ached for what would never be—my heart ached for Jenna.

The marriage reached its tipping point at that stage. Trying to hold it all together was exhausting. Trying to hold me together was even more exhausting. Jeff was adamant that we have no more children, and we fought about it every waking hour. Everything was just too much. I submissively caved into Jeff's wanting a vasectomy. He was twenty-nine, and I was thirty. It was about that time that I found wine. Not in a bad way. More in a way that when we socialized, a glass or two took the edge off. Up until that stage of life, I'd never really drank, never even been drunk at the age of thirty.

I was emotionally spent and didn't care anymore about not having any additional children with him. I didn't care to fight him. I no longer cared for him or for the marriage. I was sinking, still grieving Jenna and her twin, Julia. I needed to give her a name and place in my life as well. Life was too much; I was putting on a happy face while raising three boys and fighting postpartum depression on my own, all the while trying to plan my exit from our marriage.

Life doesn't always go as planned. We quietly, and sometimes not so quietly, verbally battled it out. Other relationships in my life, however, amounted into a "one-shot deal breaker." After I had my last son, an old friend called out of the blue. The friendship was wonderful in our early twenties, and as two newly married couples, the four of us traveled and dined together. We really enjoyed each other's company, but then it fizzled, long before my miscarriage. Jeff and I used to ask ourselves over and over what happened to our friendship with Karen and Scott. They were some of our closest friends at the time, and we missed them. The call from Karen surprised me, but I was excited to see her and hopefully mend whatever had gone wrong. She wanted to get together.

When they arrived, it was slightly uncomfortable for more than one of us. It was obvious that she was pregnant, possibly well into her fourth or fifth month with their first child. They stayed for a few hours, and before leaving, she asked to have as many baby items as she could take. Her false smile should have been the warning. I should have gone with my gut. But I didn't. I reluctantly walked her into the garage where all the boxes were neatly stacked and clearly labeled in the back corner.

I had put everything away, never parting with any of it. Just in case. In case what? I really wasn't sure. But in the back of my mind, a new narrative started.

Why did I lose Jenna?

Why didn't I get to become a mom to a girl?

Why wouldn't I ever get to be the mother of the bride?

Those narratives morphed into a new form of reasoning.

Maybe I was meant to adopt a little girl. Not everyone has the capacity to love an adopted child with all their heart just as if they had birthed them, but I knew I would love that way. Unconditional love for a child was at the core of my heart.

With that thought in mind, I shifted a few boxes marked "Give away: Baby items 0–6 months."

She glanced at them, hands on hips.

"That's it? That's all you're going to give, I mean, lend me?"

I stared at her in disbelief. This ex-friend had the nerve to call me out of the blue to only get free baby items? Not to reinvest in our friendship?

The moment of silence was broken by her huge sigh of exasperation.

"Look at all those boxes marked Jenna that you will never use. I mean, come on, don't you think you should part with them at some point? It's not like you will ever have a girl. At this point, staying married to Jeff, it's not like you will ever have any more children."

I didn't respond. It was part of a new growth pattern I was trying to establish. Not everything needed a response. I moved the chosen boxes with my foot, sliding them one at a time in her direction as the garage door opened. Jeff and his old buddy were laughing at their own happy conversation.

Karen turned to her husband.

"Pick them up, Scott. It's not like I'm in any condition to carry them. Grab the cradle as well. That's okay for us to borrow the cradle, right, Jeff?"

She stared both husbands down at the same time. Jeff's eyes darted back and forth between Karen and me; I was desperately pleading no with my eyes.

She left that day feeling slightly victorious, I would imagine. I was left feeling wounded by her words. She used my trust in her with my heartache and vulnerability as a weapon. It wasn't the first time in my life that betrayal had happened. Unfortunately, it wasn't her last go at it either.

NOTE TO SELF

Some friends and others in your life are there to teach you lessons. Some are there to stand by you through thick and thin. Some will always walk the journey and hold space for you. It takes time to figure out who is who. Sometimes you need to experience the bitter in order to appreciate the sweet. Remember the old saying, "Fool me once, shame on you; fool me twice, shame on me."

The learning experience is a balance of trusting others who show positive behavior patterns of reliability and accountability, with nonjudgmental and respectful boundaries. They are individuals who do not raise themselves up at the expense of putting another down. They do not bend over backward to please others at the expense of others and sometimes themselves. Learning to balance self-trust is honoring yourself and asking the hard question: Did I represent myself in the same manner of positive behavior?

Being able to stand up for yourself and stay true to your own truth is a major pivot in life. This sense of self, sense of strength, is one that will be tested over and over again in life, especially when you're living with chronic illness.

TAKE A MOMENT FOR YOURSELF

Breathe, Pause, Reflect . . .

Have you experienced trust issues in your life? The greatest challenges sometimes shake our vulnerability and trust.

Can you identify individuals who have shown positive behavior?

Can you match positive behavior patterns and boundaries with individuals who merit your trust and vulnerability?

Self-trust is also recognizing the balance between oversharing and being disconnected with the ability to reflect connectiveness of positive behavior. Are there positive behavior patterns in your own life that can be improved upon?

Self-authoring allows a window into oneself, be it journaling or writing. Can you see positive patterns of behavior noted?
If not, then look at the negative narrative and reflect on how it can be changed into a positive behavior pattern.

Anomalies

Never judge an individual based on their worst and best moments. These are singular anomalies, not the sum of their being.

The Brick Wall

You were not who I thought you were.
The laughter,
The sharing,
The exposed vulnerability,
A non-blooded sister bonding that should have lasted a lifetime.

You were not who I thought you were.
The supporter,
The trusted confidante,
The charismatic enigma,
A non-family family that should have lasted a lifetime.

You were not who I thought you were.
The lies,
The malice,
The hurt,
The enemy to my heart, wounding to last a lifetime.

You were not who I thought you were.
The deception,
The exposed weakness,
The lack of trust,
A catalyst to my brick wall, that will more than not last a lifetime.

CHAPTER 3

BRICK BY BRICK

Months had moved along quickly, filled with family traditions that I continued to put into place. Friday night family movie night with wings and nachos. Saturday potluck with friends. Sunday brunch of Eggs Benny followed by wonderful family dinners. Every week I planned around hockey and meals, and I always kicked it up a few notches around each holiday—filling them with decorations and making them memorable in ambiance and traditional foods that we just couldn't have a holiday without. Still to this day, Christmas just can't be Christmas without my homemade chocolate fudge.

One day, I had scheduled a playdate with my closest friend and her children. The paints were ready. The tiny sandwiches were made. Carefully decorated cookies were set out on display. I didn't bother making coffee. She lived next door, yet I knew she would make the effort to make the short drive to Tim Hortons to treat us to an extra-large double double. It was a wonderful day. We laughed so hard that we cried. The kids had a blast. The world felt right. The dark clouds of postpartum had slowly dissipated further and further apart. I waved as they left and closed the door, smiling. My house was still filled with children's laughter. I needed that day! I felt happy as I ran to pick up the ringing phone.

"Hello," I said with my voice uplifted and full of life.

"Hey, it's me, Karen. I wanted you to be the first person I called to tell you I had the baby. It's a girl. I bet you are pea-green with envy. I'm just sorry I can't see the look on your face!"

My response was simply, "Congratulations." I couldn't muster up much else. The lump in my throat was already forming, choking out anything else. I became silent, not wanting her to know she had succeeded in her final blow, her one and final shot, the deal breaker.

That moment caused extra turmoil in our marriage; Jeff said I was making a mountain out of a molehill. He insisted we go to the hospital and bring them a gift. "Don't stoop to her level; Be the bigger person; Buy them something nice for the baby, that's who we are," he said.

Begrudgingly, I walked through the baby girl section of a local store and chose a few beautiful outfits. I carefully wrapped them in lavender-colored tissues and placed them in the box. I selected a wonderful pink and lavender thick-gauge paper and folded it to perfection, taping and over taping the flaps down so they were not even visible, much like my feelings and emotions. I placed a beautiful bow on top, giving the presence of a picture-perfect happy facade, much like my fake happy face I had learned to put on.

We never had the opportunity to even see their baby. Karen accepted the gift but made excuse after excuse as to why we were not allowed to see their daughter. Seven months later, Jeff received a call to come and get the cradle. We did. Karen stayed in the house, and Scott made excuses for her. We didn't hear from them again until much later in life when they were both going through numerous pivots of their own.

NOTE TO SELF

Not everyone deserves to know your heart, the pieces that pain you.

Not everything said requires a response.

If someone wounds you deeply, take note and remember that the pain is showing you the type of behavior you do not want to repeat to another. Take in that pain, then release it as it doesn't serve you. It's a wound; make the time to heal it.

Grieving is a process. It is its own little journey and should not take up too much of your heart, your time, or space in your thoughts. Sometimes talking to a professional can make the world of difference.

Healing the wound is work. It's growth and takes time.

Plant a seed of gratitude in the right soil, nurture it, and it will grow!

TAKE A MOMENT FOR YOURSELF

Breathe, Pause, Reflect . . .

Self-authoring is a wonderful way to view our thoughts and feelings.

When you view your journal or writing, does it reflect gratitude? Is the narrative positive, reflecting a nurturing positive behavior?

If not, can you dedicate three minutes per day for three weeks prior to sleep to journal thoughts of gratitude with a positive and nurturing narrative?

Part of self-care is to nurture and protect.

Are you evenly balanced or over-weighted in a mode of self-protection?

What positive behavior patterns can you develop or implement to align yourself?

CHAPTER 4

WOMAN TO WOMAN

Life went on, and it was busy. When our older boys were young, I held down two jobs and did all the housework and most of the child rearing. That soon changed as I came to realize that I did not need to emulate past generations of motherhood. To make matters more cumbersome, I insisted on making my own baby food, as well as nursing my children longer than what the books indicated. I used cloth diapers. At that time in the '80s, these things were unfashionable. I was judged harshly by coworkers, family, and friends, all of whom seemed to be opinionated women. I called a spade a spade! The mothers who stay home judge the mothers who work, and vice versa.

Why is it that we women sometimes lack the internal fortitude to support one another?

From my experience, it was somewhat lacking. It's my opinion that it's our nature to be maternal and nurturing toward others. So why is it so difficult for some women, *mano a mano*? (This is a Spanish expression wrongfully used as "man to man" when the correct meaning is "hand to hand.") It's a form of togetherness, a united front. A joining of people, shoulder to shoulder, making us stronger. I've reflected on this entire aspect over many years, bringing in the comparison of how boys were reared when I grew up. Let's start from a basic thought. Be it a team, regiment, or brotherhood, boys generally grew up being placed in a team environment. The enemy was not other boys, but other teams. It was no different for regiments or associations. Still to this day, there is healthy rivalry among navy and army or firemen and policemen.

But women over generations have not had this bonding of team spirit. We have, however, in the past been groomed to pit one against the other. To compete singularly against each other, be it gymnastics, dance, figure skating, or beauty contests. Not only do we strive to be better than our female counterparts but also to be equally accepted by our male counterparts. An overall self-entrapment of superhero, its root quest stemming from a competitive nature and desire for equality.

And don't get me started on the "best friend" title. After my painful interaction with Karen, a former close friend—was she once a best friend?—I reflected on it. Was that the behavior I want in a close friend? No.

Some females wave the "best friend" flag around like a banner for every other female in the room to see. When was the last time you heard a man introduce himself as "Bob, Jim's best friend"? It's a myth that males are more territorial than females, especially in the friend department of life. Why do we do that? Hey, I've been guilty of it in the past. Is it that we have been so hardwired to compete against one another that we need to stake our claim: she's my best friend, go get your own? Are we that insecure? Where did that thought process start that we as females should not bond in great numbers, shoulder to shoulder? I got your back, she's got your side, we've got you covered. Was that hardwiring seed planted out of insecurity? Out of fear? If so, whose fear was it?

Sometimes we need to address the elephant in the room: insecurity. This is one of those moments that we say, "I wish I would have known then what I know now." We need to honor the strong words of "I am . . ." as in "I am good enough, just the way I am."

We doubt ourselves. We shame ourselves into believing what others think of us. We trap ourselves into caring more than we should about what others think of us, about how we project an image of oneself to our world, our family, our job, and our lifestyle. This train of thought comes with a heavy price tag. It costs some dearly, both emotionally and financially. For some, it's integrity.

Losing one's self in life's endless game of inauthenticity is time that cannot be recaptured. We all go through it to a degree. I know I did. I worked two jobs. The long hours. The loss of time with the boys and my husband left me exhausted, mentally and physically. I worked two jobs not because we needed money for food and rent. I did so because I heard several friends and family members utter criticizing words that were not encouraging, judging us as young parents and how we would never be able to provide the necessities, never mind the extras in life. The focus from others was more on what I could buy my children rather than how I would parent them and nurture them into confident human beings. It's silly now when I think of it, but again, I grew from the experience. Would I change any of it? No, because life is a journey from which we both live and learn.

Personal growth occurred over the years. The how is still a mystery to a degree, as I hadn't at that point in time really and truly grasped the depth of gratitude. It's a natural progression when life hands you lemons and you use positivity to make lemonade.

Jeff and I moved on happily. We reached a place in our marriage where we could move on together as a family. My love for Jeff, our marriage and our friendship, and our love for our boys outweighed the losses we endured.

Focusing not on what I had lost but instead on having gratitude for what I had helped the days get easier. The loss of the babies and wanting a daughter tugged at my heartstrings and popped up in the marriage from time to time, as unresolved issues do. But for the most part, we were happy. For me, the dark clouds of postpartum depression had fully lifted, as I accepted where I was in that moment in time with gratitude and made a pivot.

NOTE TO SELF

Try to be the positive female role model that you did not see represented in media, television, or the workplace. Change the narrative among females to inspire, motivate, and infuse the true power of a woman that lifts other women up, not puts them down to elevate oneself. Assertiveness and tenacity are positive attributes, so use them to lead. The depth of a true leader is to show others how great they are, not how great a leader you are!

THE BEST FRIEND

Learning to let go of what does not nurture is hard. Little did I realize that the evaluation of close friends sometimes goes in that direction, and that lesson will be repeated until it is learned. In 2015 I summed up my reflections on the topic of best friends with a post on Facebook. And it struck a nerve. It rocked the proverbial boat!

I wasn't meaning to cause such a stir . . . or was I? Truth being said, writing allows me to take all my bundled thoughts and express them. The post itself was truly just a catalyst to what I really wanted to say.

The coveted title of the "best friend" is highly overrated and gives a false sense of security. I am reflective at the moment on all my previous adult best friends. Let's face it: I'm guessing we have all had our share of who we called—and who we thought were—our best friends.

It wasn't until recently at several events that I became keenly aware of the true dynamics from my perspective of the title.

An individual at these events could not resist throwing around her "title." She constantly introduced herself this way: "Oh, hi, I'm Rita, Rosie's best friend." Then she would glance at me as if to get some reaction, for which there was none. See, I used to be Rosie's "best friend." Strange how that happens. To some attending, it wouldn't be any different from being forced to have encounters with an ex-spouse. To me, it was not relevant. At the time, I was perplexed as to why she was constantly introducing herself like that. Wrapping her identity as to project a tightly woven invisible ranking, almost desperate to unveil its cloak of invisibility to all those who she wanted and needed to witness it. I looked at Rita and noticed how her hair, her style of clothes, and even her manner had taken on the twinning of "best friend." She had lost some of her own identity as she was swept up in the relationship. I felt sad for her. I felt pity for Rita.

From my perspective, those who constantly need to use the "best friend" title are insecure in their relationship with the so-called best friend. I remember thinking to myself, Does she realize that others have held that title before her? Then I wondered if she even realized that there might, in fact, be those who will carry that title after her.

Oh, trust me, I've been there. Throwing the title around and gloating and basking in it myself. My younger self spent many wasted hours trying to figure out what went wrong with my adult best friend relationships. I spent time with a glass or two of wine in the tub when the tears just flowed into the bubbles. What went wrong? Let's be honest here. It hurts. And sometimes it wounds so deeply that we never want to go back there again.

There's a lightbulb moment when you realize you didn't really mean that much to them. Or should I say that you invested more in the relationship than they did. Or is it something more profound? Have we learned what was needed from the depth of that friendship and therefore no longer nurtured each other's growth? Whatever the way, when a best friend relationship goes south, we grieve for what was and for the moments that have yet to be.

People use excuses as to why the relationship ended. They will falsely tag the loss of relationship on a move, a divorce, or a change in work to paint the dotted line to a reason. The truth is that they just stopped trying, and the pivots of time went in different directions. The best friend relationship is no different from any other relationship. It takes two to make it work and two to keep it going. For some, these friends are nothing more than a stepping-stone to either growth or regression. Yes, regression. I have watched in complete shock at how some regress to be torn down, which then allowed them to be rebuilt, while I, with hands tied, watched from the sidelines. That's life.

Sometimes the relationship ends with a verbal knock-down fight with everything going down in flames, other times it fizzles like a candle that slowly burns out over time, its wick eventually coming to an end. I'm not sure which is worse, as I have only experienced the wick running out in several adult best friend relationships. Either way, it still burns. In my experience, it will only burn as long as you allow it to. Personally, I wouldn't have it any other way. I am truly thankful for my ex-best friends as I now look back, laugh, and fondly remember good times. I can easily walk into a room, give them a hug, and move on. I know with others, the wick is still there, possibly waiting to be fanned when older, wiser women have realized what was truly lost: a bond of trust, love, and loyalty like grains of sand escaping through our fingers. The life lessons that an ex-best friend has given me are pivotal moments in time that have allowed me to have profound personal growth as an individual. Through those lessons, I have taught myself that forgiveness is something one does for one's self. I have learned that the true "best friend" is the one who is there through thick and thin and doesn't feel necessary to flaunt the fake title because they know who they are. We work at it, and because its reciprocal, we feel it.

For all those who have best friends, take heart, care, and love. Be trustworthy and invest deeply because in the end, you will either be the "best friend" (title not required), or their loss—the "best friend" who got away!

TAKE A MOMENT FOR YOURSELF

Breathe, Pause, Reflect . . .

Do you carry the title of best friend?

Do you think as a narrative that it matters?

Would the change in narrative make a difference?

"Hi, I'm Rita, Rosie's best friend." (Best being #1, first place, a title, territorial)
"Hi, I'm Rita. Nice to meet you. How long have you known Rosie? We've been close friends for twenty years now." (No title, not territorial, explains the depth of their relationship because they worked on it. Open-ended and inclusive, as many people can have a close relationship when it is mutually worked on.)

CHAPTER 5

THE COFFEE TRUCK DRIVER'S WIFE

1996–2000

It was, for the most part, a freezing cold day. A leap year: February 29. It was also memorable, as we moved into the crappiest house on the street. I had waited patiently over six months for the price to drop. The house had been on my radar since fall when the grass was so long that one of the neighbors had called the city to come and cut it. We had bought a Power of Sale house in one of the nicest of neighborhoods. Honestly, we were as proud as could be, coming from very humble beginnings. We had family, however, who were overwhelmed by looking at the fixer-upper and even cried at our "diamond in the rough," as they could not see past the work to be done and the mess that was in front of their eyes. The last owners left in an angry haste. Drywall was punched in numerous spots, and the living room carpet had been stained from end to end with what looked to be an entire pot of coffee and needed immediate removal.

I stood there in the drive, surveying the street. I didn't know the names of the people who were my neighbors, but I did know some of their professions: doctors, lawyers, teachers, dentists, real estate brokers, and CEOs. They didn't know me either. But as time passed, I was simply referred to as "the coffee truck driver's wife."

I stood there grinning from ear to ear. Plenty of room for the boys. Plenty of growth potential in the property. From both the logical side of my brain and my heart, it had been a great buy. Location, location, location.

I had always been good with money and with numbers. Several generations before me had lived through the Depression and some, two wars. I learned very early the value of a hard-earned dollar, how to pinch pennies, and how to make one chicken stretch into three meals: chicken dinner, chicken pot pie, and chicken soup. It came in handy when I was first married. We literally held regular card games with friends so I could cash in the beer bottles to buy bread and milk.

Our youngest was four when we moved into the crappiest

house on the nicest street. I had just started back to work in the banking world. It was a major bank on the wealth management side. After securing my position, I took advantage of advancing my education. The bank paid as long as I passed, which seemed like a win-win from my perspective.

My choice to pivot was out of need. I needed to move on after the postpartum depression. I needed to put more time and energy into my own personal growth. I also needed to be the breadwinner that had added perks of stock-buying plans and, most importantly, family benefits. It needed to be on me if our family wanted to live the lifestyle we wanted to carve out.

Jeff is the hardest working man I have ever known in my life. He's dedicated and never takes a day off. He has dyslexia and has run and operated a coffee truck all his life. My own drive and dedication to education and work ethics paid off, as I continued to push myself to be more knowledgeable in the male-dominated field. I obtained my CSC (Canadian Securities Course), CPH (Conduct Practices Handbook), PFP (Professional Financial Planning), and LLQP (Life License Qualification Program). I also completed my Mortgage Agents License Certification.

It was a hard go to forge through what was known as "the Boys' Club." Even with my credentials, I was hit with the reality that when men outside the firm were being hired as wealth advisers, they had less education and experience than I did. I took a giant leap, with my assertiveness in check, and pushed myself directly in management's path to be acknowledged in my field. At first, they pushed back. I remember a smug manager saying to me, "You're a great senior broker's assistant. Why don't you just stick to what you're good at?"

Well, that only made me want to push, and push hard! With all my facts ready (the names of all the new male hires and a list of their credentials or lack thereof), I presented my case. My key sentence was that the outside hires being all male and not specifically qualified seemed discriminatory to the females within the firm who were overqualified. Discriminatory. Yes, I played that card, as frankly, it was appropriate. What mattered to the bank was that they brought with them a small book of business. That said, the up-and-coming female advisers should have been given the opportunity to purchase a small book of business to get started.

My assertiveness, credentials, work ethic, and grit paid off. I was promoted to a wealth adviser. My pivot was in full force. I opened a door for myself into the "club" and prepared to break that glass ceiling—and break it, I would! It also helped create opportunities for other women in the firm to follow suit. But this leap didn't come without challenges. Life itself doesn't come without challenges and growth. Throughout my career as a wealth adviser, I encountered sexist comments, harassment, and bullying. That is where some individuals' mindsets were at. I chose to brush off those minefields and focus on the positives about my career and industry. With my title and credentials in hand, I strived to service my clients both morally and ethically. I loved the industry back then. What I cherished the most was being of service to my clients.

Careers, like other things in life, can sometimes be invisible to the outside world. All that education and knowledge, yet my neighbors still referred to me as "the coffee truck driver's wife." I laugh at it to this day. In reality, it was nothing more than the neighbors not being aware of my career and more about a marker as to where we lived. The "marker" was gleaming and pretty unmistakable. If you looked down our street, you would see the driveways lined with car after car until you got to ours. In its shining glory with glistening chrome, a large coffee truck was parked in our driveway. I was just as proud of that truck as my husband. He was self-employed, and I managed the bookkeeping when he first started out up until he semiretired at fifty. When he started his career in the industry, business was booming; however, at the end of his career, the coffee truck industry was a dinosaur. Every corner had a coffee shop, fast food place, or a gas station with all of them together, one "stop and shop." Frankly, it was Jeff's time to pivot.

As an adviser, the days were long when I was building my book of business, as it was called. My client base was filled with individuals of varying backgrounds and ages. My briefcase was a testament to that, always filled with handouts that referred to specific investment strategies and suggestions.

I was always overly prepared and had ample handouts. At the end of my day, my briefcase was just as full as when the day started. I exited my "mom van," making the small walk to the mailbox with my briefcase weighing me down. My intent was to grab the mail and head to the house to prep dinner for the family. Yes, I wore more than one hat, and at all times, I might add. It made me who I was: an adviser with empathy for a growing family or a retired couple. It didn't matter who they were, I invested as if it were my own money, basing it on age, value, safety, and quality.

The evening was just as any other day of the week when it started. My briefcase just as heavy, keys to the mailbox fumbling in my hand as I tried to retrieve the letters and loads of junk mail from the ever-so-small box. Turning quickly, I almost ran over one of my neighbors. She smiled at me and said, "You're the coffee truck driver's wife, aren't you?"

I smiled back and said, "Yes, yes, I am." My reply sounded much like a chuckle.

"I'm Sue. What is it that you do for a living?"

I stretched out my hand to shake and replied, "I'm Anne Marie; I'm a wealth adviser."

"Oh," she said, almost shocked. "Good for you! There must not be many females in your position?"

I shook my head, as it was true. I said my goodbyes and turned to go.

My mind flashed to my work life. I was, for the most part, working in a sea of male advisers. Walking back to the house, I recalled my first day at a convention at the Royal York in Toronto. I'd always loved that hotel. I could not have chosen a better spot for my first experience being away from Jeff and the boys. I could not have imagined a better spot to imprint a memory of a glorious and triumphant moment in time. It seemed like as if it were yesterday. I had donned my best power suit, in red. Heels, check. Coordinated purse, check. Accessories, check. Confidence, check and check! I opened those double doors to the convention as proud as I could be. I walked into the disproportionately weighted male crowd of blue and black suits as if my red suit was saying, "I'm here and bloody well get used to it! And by the way, get ready because I'm going to be assisting in recruiting and mentoring future female advisers."

When I first started out as an adviser, I was full of excitement and ambition, and it became part of the fabric of my being, part of my identity. I was intrinsically linked to it. I worked hard and against the odds and still succeeded. Like a character in a play, I dressed the part. Acted the part. Lived the part and loved the part. It was without a doubt rewarding emotionally and financially. I felt accomplished and confident, and because I was fully accredited, it was justified. Every once in a while, I felt this twinge of mild anxiety that everyone was going to figure out I was not worthy of this role as an adviser to be trusted with millions and millions of the bank's and clients' money.

Impostor syndrome is a common term used to describe the experience of the self-doubt of one's abilities, as well as the feeling of being somewhat like a fraud more than not in the work environment. The term is generally given to women and minorities, basically those who do not fit into society's stereotypes. It's not a formal diagnosis, and using the term is problematic in itself. The feeling (an experience) of being an impostor for most stems from an overall universal feeling of unease, anxiety, and self-doubt due to systemic effects in the workplace and society. It generally affects individuals who are high achievers who break the social boundaries of a set role. They edge their way into a non-inclusive environment. The problem isn't the so-called impostor, it's the lack of the workplace environment producing a multitude of role models and leaders diverse in gender and ethnicity. All professionals within a field of choice should feel that their workplace fosters an inclusive environment.

I was a woman walking in what generations before me (and some present) said were "men's shoes." It was a thought that became more than prevalent as my career ended. I began to feel somewhat defeated by a bully who went out of his way to make me feel inferior, especially once I was dealing with chronic illness.

Our boys, our marriage, and my career all thrived. My career opened a whole new lifestyle that I had never dreamed of. We regularly vacationed as a family, sometimes just Jeff and me, and sometimes with friends. We fine-dined and entertained every weekend. We explored; travel, food, and wine were my main joys when the boys were grown. It was the first time in our marriage that financial stress had been lifted. We had spent approximately twenty years living week to week, paycheck to paycheck. I finally felt this heavy burden lifted when I was in control of my income and felt compelled to carefully implement financial goals that included helping the boys by paying for their education. We were also able to tuck a set amount away for each to gift later on in life when they would start out on their own journey of possibly buying a home or traveling.

I was never able to give up a good hat, meaning as a woman, my shirt, like all multitasking women, should have read "superwoman." I had to do it all, be the best I could be at it all. I shifted hats with ease, from adviser hat to mom hat to spouse hat to daughter, sister, aunt, friend, neighbor, and service to community hat. I loved my mom hat by far the most. As life moved on, I realized that some of the hats worn were not appreciated or reciprocated. I felt I was always the one giving and putting effort into the relationships. I made a note of it at the time but did nothing else. When exhausted, I would sit in a quiet room with a glass or two of my favorite red and my Yorkies, who were always wanting to snuggle and listen. My dogs never judged and always made me feel loved and filled with joy. Reflecting on my wonderful family, as busy as it was, also always filled me with love and gratitude.

I led a charmed life. One that my unplanned pivot had given me. You see, I hadn't planned on being a wealth adviser. But the opportunities opened, and the tides changed, so I went with the tide. The unexpected shift in direction had led to this point in time. It was a gift the universe had given to me. Or did I create the gift for myself? I never once gave thought to there ever being any other pivots in life before or after that moment in time. After all, life was somewhat linear, right?

NOTE TO SELF

If given an opportunity to learn and grow, but you fall . . . rise, get up, and just keep moving forward.

Pivots in life are what we make of them. The direction isn't as important as your attitude and mindset.

TAKE A MOMENT FOR YOURSELF

Breathe, Pause, Reflect . . .

Do you identify with your job or career of choice?

How does it reflect your personality?

Have you ever experienced impostor syndrome?

What did you implement to move forward from the experience?

Did you choose your career or job, or did it choose you?

What did you want to be as a child?

Does your career or job match what you wanted as a child?

Did you relate happiness as a child to your chosen decision of what you wanted to be when you grew up?

Happiness is a state of mind. It also brings joy. It is limitless. What brought you joy as a child?

The Gift of Joy

She gave of herself, the beauty
that filled her eyes,

She gave of herself, the treasures
that filled her senses,

She gave of herself, the whimsy
that filled her mind,

She gave of herself, the prized belongings
that filled her life,

She gave of herself, the art of giving
that filled her heart.

Dedicated to: Marion Gordon Adney
(Beloved Nana)

CHAPTER 6

MONARCH BUTTERFLY

2006

I sat pensive, staring at the gravestone. I ran my fingers across the engraved name and date, its crevices deeper than the eyes could see, much like the wounds to my heart. I am generally a stoic individual. I'm the "fall down, brush yourself off, and get back up" kind of woman. I will admit, sometimes I'm down much longer than I will ever show. This time, life had punched me and our extended family in the gut, taking the wind out of our lungs and wounding our hearts in different and sometimes unspeakable ways. Each of us was going on our own journey because death created a pivotal moment in time, and for many, we went in completely different directions.

We've all heard a version of this before, and here's mine: The wounded bleed all over everyone else if they don't heal. And if you don't heal what hurt you, you'll bleed on people who didn't cut you.

My older sister, Nancy Jean, passed away on July 8, 2006, a few months after turning fifty-two, after a long and courageous battle with lung cancer. I say long, but the time passed in a blur, and sometimes, selfishly, I feel it passed too quickly but also not quickly enough in the end.

I am not a stranger to death. As a family, we had a string of deaths prior, all within five years of one another. My father passed away in 2001, and his brother Herman just weeks before. I felt very differently about those two deaths. I grieved for my father when Alzheimer's left him as an empty shell of a man waiting in limbo for peace at the end of his journey. I was as ready as one could be. But I did have unanswered questions about his life.

My therapist asked me how I reacted to his death.

I thought to myself, *what a weird question.* In reality, it was a great question. I had to dig deep and be honest. My reaction to his death was one of acceptance and relief.

"Did you cry?"

Again, I needed to be authentic. My response was honest. I

cried at the funeral, more so because of watching others in their grieving process. I cried as I grieved his loss when Alzheimer's hit. I visited him briefly when he was in an extended-care facility. I visited him alone, and my visits felt partly due to a childlike love and obligation. They weighed heavily on me emotionally, then physically in the end for several reasons. The care facility was a brown-brick four-story building that lacked appeal. Its entrance wasn't adorned with flowers or greetings. It could have been any commercial-type building, bland and lacking in personality. The hospital-like flooring gave hint to its purpose. The elevator didn't give away anything at the first floor, but as it rose to the upper locked areas of the facility, the smell of urine mixed with bleach was overwhelming. When the doors opened, you were greeted with a lineup of elderly strapped into wheelchairs. Some were happy to see a new face, others stared off into the abyss. Signing in was mandatory and routine. The update on where he was in the moment was also routine.

"Unresponsive" was generally the update. I had been going for visits over a period of time, and nothing had changed.

"He won't recognize you. He doesn't recognize his surroundings either," the attendant said with an empathetic smile.

I put my sweatshirt sleeve up to my nose. I had learned to spray a bit of perfume on the cuff, so I could block out the urine smell in order to tolerate any quick visit without vomiting. The perfume made me dizzy and gave me a headache, but it did the trick.

I made my way down the narrow pathway with wheelchairs flanking me on both sides. I tried to look and smile and keep moving as fast as I could. Halfway down to his room, I passed the TV room on my left and paused to notice several men and women strapped in their wheelchairs and watching a show. As I turned to continue, there seemed to be a commotion, the sound of grunting becoming louder and louder and frantic in nature. I paused again to walk back to the TV room.

My eyes looked at the grunting man, his voice becoming quieter as I closed in. His frail body looked emaciated and lost within the bulky fabric of his pajamas. His blue eyes unmistakably my father's. I brushed the wisp of hair on top of his head.

He knew it was me, or he at least knew it was someone he recognized. In the beginning, when he was first taken to the facility, he called me Lorette, his sister's name. When he did so, it was sad but validated where he was in that moment in time. I had to fight the urge to correct him and sadly responded anyway. On this day, I didn't care. I would have been happy if he smiled and called me Lorette; I would have gladly played a part for the few moments before it was taken away. I was just happy I caught him in a moment when he had some recognition. I dragged a visitor's chair along the sterile 1950's flooring. Its pinks, greens, yellows, and blues giving the only dim pop of color to the beige life in the room.

I sat next to my father in hopes of having a conversation that could hint at his recognition of who I was. Instead, he turned away from me. His grunting ceased. His hand slowly reached to the back of his shirt where he tried to flip the edge up. He became slightly agitated, so I leaned in to quietly ask him what he was doing. Before I got the opportunity, he put his hand gently on mine and pulled it to his back, flipping his pajama shirt up. Then, in that moment, I realized he knew who I was. He wanted me to scratch his back as I had done so many times as a child. I obliged; he smiled. During the back scratch, he quietly and forever drifted to the abyss and never returned to a moment of recognition.

I visited a few times after that. Then I didn't. I had to stop as the emotional and physical exhaustion was taking its toll. I grieved and said my goodbyes long before his physical passing.

I had already moved on, so his physical death became closure. I was in full acceptance of his passing. The shell or vessel had gone to join the man.

My father and my Uncle Herman looked like twins to a degree, just fourteen months apart at birth. They passed away three weeks apart. Herman left this world slightly before my father, just how he had entered this world slightly earlier than my father had.

Herman's death was a different story from my father's; he'd had a quick, aggressive cancer. I was very attached to my uncle. He had stepped forward in my father's Alzheimer's absence. He was fully invested in his role as a dual uncle and father figure. He was loving, supportive, caring and funny, and he called a spade a spade. I loved all those qualities about him. When he passed, it was sudden. I felt angry and selfishly ripped off from having him in my life in this role for what seemed like a moment. He filled this void for which I didn't recognize there was such a hole in my heart to be filled. The time was just too short for his parental love. Forever and always his Rosebud.

My sister Nancy's passing seemed a combination of both types of grieving at first. However, I didn't anticipate its depth and duration. I didn't anticipate the guilt I would feel from the hopes and wishes I couldn't keep due to illness and life itself. I didn't anticipate the gap she would leave in the birthing order. I didn't anticipate the void she would leave, nor the wound that failed to heal for many within our family. I didn't anticipate that it would happen so suddenly that I could barely catch my breath. And I truly didn't anticipate my stoic demeanor unraveling like a thread on the hem of a dress.

It was so long ago, yet it feels as if it were yesterday. The call came as a shock. Nancy had seemed stable the night before. In fact, she had seemed like she had had a burst of energy.

The voice at the other end of the phone seemed to echo and reverberate off my eardrum. "You better come now if you want to say goodbye."

Frantically, I made a few phone calls. One to a family member in which I let her know my father-in-law would pick her up, then we would meet and I would drive to Sudbury to say our goodbyes. It was all a blur, the phone call, the drive up. I did so in disbelief. I had spoken to her the night before. We talked and watched *Jeopardy* together, playing along as she kicked my ass. She laughed at my lack of knowledge, then she filled me in on her advantage: her feed of TV was slightly faster than mine, so she knew the answers in advance of me. I still laugh at that. She had been happy, comfortable, and positive the night before. Yet there I was, driving the next day to say goodbye.

I remember walking as fast as I could into the hospital. The elevator ride up seemed too slow, and the hallway seemed too long. Walking into her hospital room, I could hear the machines slowly beeping. There were tubes and trays all around Nancy, who lay peacefully in the crisp cotton sheets. Her tiny figure seemed childlike and peaceful. Cancer is a beast, but she kept trying to slay it right until her last breath. I gave hugs around the room. We chatted about nothing, anything. We all walked the journey, but in our own ways. Some left later in the day, some stayed. Some showered and ate, some did not.

I stayed. I would do my best to hold myself together and wait it out. I touched her arms, held her hand, spoke to her softly. I patted her tiny feet. They were cold, so I carefully placed her fuzzy socks on her and tightly wrapped the blanket all around her body, tucking her in.

Those of us who stayed took turns going to the bathroom and grabbing snacks and drinks, not wanting to leave her alone.

When I was alone with her, I took my time to say my goodbyes out loud. Holding her hand, I asked her not to fight it anymore. I whispered that she deserved peace from the torment, peace from the pain. I told her to go be the monarch butterfly she promised me she would morph in to. I leaned into her and gave her butterfly kisses on her nose and whispered, "I got this. You know you can trust that I got this. Go be a butterfly in peace. I will always watch and wait for you. Promise me you will find me."

The hours continued, and we waited as her breath became staggered and raspy, then we waited some more. The daytime light blurred into nighttime darkness.

It was hard to watch, hard to bear, hard to hear, hard to let go. But let go, we did. It was blatantly obvious to all that the pain medication wasn't enough. She was horribly uncomfortable. The nurses offered to change her position. They also let us know that a change of position could sometimes result in a quicker passing.

Those of us who stood in the hall between the cold hospital walls made the unanimous decision to change her position to make her more comfortable. We all sat around her bed and tearfully watched and listened as she fought her last breaths. There was nothing to do but hold her hand. I looked down at her tiny hand in mine, her skin so thin that each vein was pronounced like ripples of blue water over pale sands. I tried to focus on being in the moment, creating peace and comfort as she passed on. I listened intently to the rhythm of her breathing, the gurgle getting louder and slower. I sat waiting for her next breath, waiting until there was no more. No more pain, no more torment, sadly, no more life to be had. She passed in the wee hours of the morning on July 8. Time stood still but for a moment.

I felt numb. I had been up for more than twenty-four hours when I chose to drive myself the four-hour trip home. I barely even remember the drive. I showered and changed and popped over to the neighbor's fiftieth birthday party. The balloons, the wine, the appetizers, the music seemed fittingly unfitting. The world just goes on, doesn't it? My husband and boys were there, waiting and expecting me. I said my hellos and gave my "happy birthday" hugs, all while wearing my fake smile mask of "I'm good." I proceeded to down a glass of red and take a small nibble of an appetizer in an effort to participate. Making no eye contact, I slowly exited the neighbor's yard and quietly and numbly walked across the street to our house where I fell into bed fully clothed. I gripped the pillow, pressing it tightly over my face to drown out my screams and to sop up my tears. I reassured myself then, and my husband later that evening, that I was okay. That I was fine. "I'm good. I got this," I said.

The next morning, Jeff picked up coffee and donuts, making my morning transition easier. I sat quietly most of the day and evening. Again, reassuring myself and my husband that I was alright. "I got this," I said, with a fake plaster smile.

Monday had arrived, and the day started off at the usual quick pace. Lunches to make, kids to drop off, briefcase to arrange, and calls to organize. With the kids gone, the house was quiet, and I had time for coffee and a few business calls. I felt like a work-from-home day was the best decision. I filled the coffee in the brewer. It smelled good and looked deeply rich against the white filter holder. I turned it on and placed my favorite mug on the counter. There was a day-old donut forgotten in the box that was tossed on top of the microwave. I took a huge bite, the hardened icing and sweetness paining me. I brushed off the sprinkles and looked at the donut, half gone with one bite, my teeth impression leaving a savage attack on its round perfection.

Just then, my ears picked up a horrific, familiar noise. It was a gurgle, then louder and more random, spewing and struggling to gurgle on. I turned and ran toward it, my heart beating as if I could be there to catch her last breath again. I stood there staring at the coffee maker, full and on its last gurgle, steam pushing out its last drop, its last breath. With tears streaming down my face, I grabbed the entire glass pot and flung it into the stainless sink, coffee and glass going in every direction. Not missing a beat, I snatched up the coffee maker with both hands and yanked the cord from the wall in one swift movement. I stormed to the garage door and heaved the coffee maker over my head to the floor. As if that wasn't enough to destroy it, I proceeded to beat it to death with a hockey stick while yelling, "I GOT THIS!" over and over until the words were but a whisper and the stick was broken. Shards of broken plastic and metal were strewn all over the concrete floor, forever fragmented, much like my heart in that moment.

Slumping to the garage floor in emotional and physical exhaustion, I gave the coffee maker one last glare and angry warning as the tears streamed down my cheeks: "Don't mess with a hockey mom."

Hours later, I was composed, and the mess was cleaned up. After all, "I got this."

Weeks later, my sister's burial, on a very hot summer's day, brought a bit more closure. We all traveled to Britt, a small town in Northern Ontario, as it was Nancy's choice of where to be buried. It was fitting. She loved "God's country," as we all called it. She's in the same graveyard where our paternal grandparents are buried, as well as some extended family, including our Uncle Raymond who never made it to his second birthday after choking on a cookie. She is surrounded by family in an area that felt like home to her. With clean blue waters and tall, lush pines, the location is nature at its best.

The motel where I was staying was anything but that. It was very clean but dated. It had a small-town vibe, and it worked. The window air conditioning unit was humming at full crank, and the room smelled a bit musty. I wondered how long it'd been since the filter had been changed in it.

It was a super-hot weekend, and my face was scarlet, the way it always is in the heat. But I wasn't sweating. Over the past few months, I had grown into a non-sweater, which seemed odd to me. How could I just not sweat? It didn't seem normal, and I had brought it up in several appointments with my doctor. And there I was, standing at the graveside with about thirty others in the sweltering heat, and I was the only one with a bright red face who wasn't sweating. Those around me were sweating profusely, wiping their faces and dabbing their tears away from their eyes. When it was over, some walked off to eat and drink. I, however, needed the bathroom in ways that I didn't realize at the time would become a routine.

I rushed to the bathroom, dragging my legs as if each one weighed 400 pounds. I barely reached the toilet, not knowing which end to put down first. I grabbed the garbage can just in case it decided to come up rather than down. Once done, I slid to the bathroom floor, placing my burning face to the cool tiles. *What the hell brought that on?* I thought to myself. As quick as it came on, it was gone. Yet my legs still felt heavy, I still felt flushed, my heart was beating frantically, and I still wasn't sweating.

I lay there on the motel bathroom floor, tracing the grout lines with my fingers to distract me from my racing heartbeat. *It's nothing serious*, I reassured myself. *It'll go away.* Turning my head over so the other cheek could feel the cool tiles, my logical mind went into reality mode. If I was really being honest with myself, I hadn't been feeling well for months. I'd been dragging my ass since I fell ill with a viral infection a few months prior. To top it off, a weekend getaway up in Moon River in May had left me with deerfly bites on my ankles, which swelled up like balloons. I ended up at an emergency clinic from the bites. It looked like I had painted on bright blush-red from mid-foot to mid-calf. They burned and were hot to the touch. A long round of antibiotics was prescribed. All seemed well on the surface after that, yet between the viral infection and the bites, I'd never quite felt the same. I blamed the exhaustion on work and the lack of sleep that came from my mind waiting until 2 a.m. to run its own narrative on various topics.

I'm sure it will pass, I reasoned. After all, I'd rarely been sick in the past.

NOTE TO SELF

It's okay to not be okay!

Allow yourself the same grace you would gladly give to others. Allow yourself to grieve fully in all its raw, unbridled emotions. Even the strongest of individuals need a shoulder to cry on or a longer hug than usual. It's not a sign of weakness—it's human nature. Allow your vulnerability and your needs to be known by those you can trust with your heart.

TAKE A MOMENT FOR YOURSELF

Breathe, Pause, Reflect . . .

Have you lost a loved one?

How did it make you grow as an individual?

When you talk about the loss, do you talk from the wound or from the scar?

The wound refers to trauma that is still painful and raw and needs some time before it can mend.

The scar refers to some healing, even if it's ugly, that has taken place.

I found that at this stage of life, I wish I would have realized that it's okay to not be okay. That it's alright to "not have this." But admitting we are not okay can be a struggle. Faking that we are fine is much harder on us overall.

Tears

Where do tears come from?
They seem to flow from the heart,

For joy, happiness, and sorrow,
all three will make them start.

I won't waste my tears on heartache,
as I know they flow in vain.

I will fill my life with tears of joy
until we meet again.

Dedicated to:

Nancy Jean Godin
April 8, 1954–July 8, 2006

CHAPTER 7

THE PERFECT STORM

2007

Weeks rolled into months after my sister Nancy passed away. I busied myself with work, kids, and friends. Jeff and I had purchased our first cottage the year earlier, so I kept myself overly busy with the plans for the renovation. I kept plugging along in life as if all was okay. It was on the surface, yet I still had horrible GI issues, wasn't sweating, and had bouts of brain fog and horrible tachycardia. My family doctor referred me to a cardiologist, who ordered a halter-monitor to track my rapid heartbeat. He put my bouts of tachycardia down to stress. "Nothing to worry about. It will pass," he said.

But was it just stress? Just nerves? Would it pass as he assured me?

It was a momentous milestone for Jeff and me in 2007 as we celebrated our twenty-fifth wedding anniversary. We were going to treat ourselves to a two-week all-inclusive vacation in the Dominican Republic at a five-star resort. It had all the bells and whistles, and we were so looking forward to the getaway. It was worked hard for and well deserved.

I looked at my Day-Timer schedule loaded with sticky notes and highlighted dates, florescent in all their glory. Everything was so neatly color-coded. Blue for the boys, #1, #2, #3, according to birthing order; yellow for business-related appointments and meetings; pink for friends and the entertaining schedule; orange for . . . hmm. I looked at the orange highlighted day. It was the only orange in the month. I had almost forgotten that my gastro-enterologist had booked me in for a colonoscopy and endoscopy.

Tapping my pen rapidly, I thought to myself, *Shit, what was I thinking, trying to fit this in between two busy workdays? Not to mention me agreeing that if they were going in to have a look they might as well get me from both ends.*

It took every ounce of restraint to not pick up the phone to cancel. I didn't have time for it. I didn't want to be laid up for a day. I had so much business to attend to and kids' things to organize before I headed off on a much-needed vacation. I looked at the requisition that was paper clipped to the backside of the Day-Timer. It needed to be done. Besides, I might drop five to eight pounds just taking the prep. Everyone could benefit from a great cleanout every once in a while. The appointment stayed in the schedule. I begrudgingly reminded myself that my favorite foods weren't sitting right in my stomach and that I was eating antacids like candy.

I remembered one incident: it was an anomaly, so I will call it a one-time event. It was just like any other day. My GI issues hadn't changed much. Food wouldn't stay in long enough to digest. After eating, my stomach muscles would stiffen like a ball and become painful. Having gone through delivery of three children, I can only describe the stomach pain as similar. My stomach would contract and remain contracted for hours. It was visible to the eye and hard to the touch. This happened on the regular, but this one day, it added a twist. I was working at my desk in the basement, relaxed in the chair while reading an article online. I suddenly felt an inner vibration. It built and built in strength, then as if someone had grabbed my intestines from end to end, it shook violently. I stood up in shock. By the time I made my way up the six steps to the family room, it was gone. It had stopped abruptly. It was if my entire intestinal tract went into spasms. It was the first and only time this happened, for which I'm thankful. I made a note to tell the GI specialist about the event.

The day for looking at me inside out from both ends crept up on me like a sneaky cat. Silently, quickly, then pounce. I was downing the prep and water like a champ. Maybe not quite a champ, more like a trouper. Smile on and limited gagging. I waited patiently in nothing but my robe, steps from the toilet. It began with a wave and ended with a tsunami. Keeping my fluids up wasn't difficult, as I was always thirsty and drank lots of water every day. I crawled into bed and hoped for a restful sleep before the peekaboo procedure. Jeff and I chatted about the trip, the boys, and relaxed while watching a bit of TV before calling it a night.

Suddenly I sat upright in bed and felt waves of panic wash over me. Looking at Jeff, I jumped out of bed and gripped the comforter as I leaned in and looked at him with pleading eyes.

"I don't feel well, I don't feel well. Oh, God, I don't feel well." This was the first time I had used that sentence. Unfortunately, it would not be the last time.

I couldn't express exactly what the feeling of unwell actually meant. It was horribly foreign to me. I had a sense of dread, as if I was going to die. I've had anxiety and a panic attack before. That's not what this was. This was a whole new level of not feeling well.

Jeff urged me to crawl back into bed and assured me that I was going to be fine. I lay there quietly as my body began to betray me. I was terrified as ripples of fasciculation started in my thighs, then moved to my torso. I shook violently. My head snapped back as my teeth chattered so hard that they chipped. I stuttered and my arms shook wildly. Five minutes in, it stopped as quickly as it had started. I lay there motionless. I was fully aware of my surroundings, fully aware during and after. I had a sudden urge to pee and rushed to the toilet. My legs felt like jelly, and I used any and every wall to balance my way to the seat.

What the fuck was that? What just happened? It was a horrible experience, one that I hoped would never happen again. You know what they say, you can hope on one hand and shit that happens in the other, guess what fills up first? Yup, shit that happens!

The actual GI scopes were uneventful, as were the results. I was clean as a whistle and ready to jet off to the Dominican for a much-needed vacay!

The night of the "attack," as I named it, was behind me, two weeks earlier. It was an anomaly, right?!

What I needed was sun, surf, food, booze, and some TLC with one of my favorite humans, my person. It was the first time we had done two weeks away from the kids, from work, and from Canada, for that matter, since our honeymoon twenty-five years prior.

Pulling up on the tarmac at the Dominican airport in 2007 was an unforgettable experience. I was filled with awe over the lush tropical greens as I peeked out the window before we disembarked. The doors opened and a gush of unbearable heat filled the cabin. The air was so humid, I could hardly breathe. We walked directly off the plane onto the tarmac, my eyes focusing on each step in front of me, only looking up to glance at my husband's back as his golf shirt started to cling to his damp body. Once my feet were on solid ground, I lifted my head and took in my surroundings. My smile faded quickly as I assessed the line of armed men that surrounded one end of the tarmac. We were greeted inside and assured it was a typical landing, a typical day at the Dominican airport. I still felt very uneasy about the number of armed men required to start off a relaxing vacation. It didn't sit right with me. We had traveled to other countries and had never experienced that type of greeting before. It was unnerving, frightening, and a very unwelcome party.

We proceeded to our resort without issues, and it was as advertised: lush, tropical, welcoming. It was our own little fantasy island. The beach with its white sands and teal blue ocean was just what I needed. It was time to unwind and focus on just the two of us. The food was great, the booze was plentiful, and there was lots to do, or not to do. Options are always good. We waded through the huge pool toward the swim-up bar while Caribbean music played in the background. Life was good. I looked in the opposite direction of the bar and noticed a man on a hanging scaffold with a sprayer. I cocked my head while shielding my eyes to see more clearly.

"What is that guy doing?" I asked the bartender.

"Oh, he's spraying off all the black mold that gets on the

hotels." His tone was casual and relaxed, as it was a common occurrence that happened at the resort.

I shrugged, sipped on my drink, and went on with my second day.

Jeff and I have always been structured kind of people. Even away from home, we seemed to fall into a routine while vacationing, getting up around the same time and easing into our morning with coffee and pastries. Then we'd take turns jetting to the ocean to drop off our towels and beach items. We did the same just before lunch when we would see two loungers available together near the pool; we would mark our seats, enjoy lunch, and hang by the pool until the pre-dinner hour. It was a great little routine, and we were having a wonderful time—until we weren't.

Only a few days into our vacation, I felt ill. Dizzy. I had a bit of a rash from the sun, I was told by the doctor at the on-site clinic. My lips were slightly swollen and my face a bit puffy, as if allergic. I was incredibly foggy, almost like I was drugged or drunk. I showered for dinner anyway, peeling off my bandage from my two toes where I'd developed blisters after wearing new sandals on a long walk the day before. We had trudged through the busy small town to view the shops and sites. Our feet got wet from an open urinal outhouse that was placed on the cobblestone walkway. Many men were using it to make room for more beer. It was funny at the time. But not so funny in the days to come once we looked back on it.

I stood there in the shower as the cool water hit my face, hoping it would snap me out of my haze. The water beaded on my suntanned and oiled skin.

Come on, Anne Marie, get your shit together. This is no time to get sick, I said to myself.

At this point, we were only five days into our fourteen-day vacation. I dressed and reassured Jeff that I was good to go.

"Let's do this," I said with a smile as we headed off for drinks and dinner.

The evening was uneventful. We had a good time and headed up to call it a night. I looked at our lovely room and smiled—our bed was made, and we had fresh flowers from the staff.

We crawled into bed, and the cool cotton sheets felt wonderful against our warm skin. The ceiling fan hummed at full force. It felt like we had only been sleeping for a few hours when I sat upright in bed. I reached over and clicked on the light while shaking Jeff with my other hand. He looked at me as my face and neck started to contort and every muscle in my body contracted tightly, on and off. I went into panic mode as I bolted from bed to the full-length mirror. I stood there gripping the night table as I looked at myself in horror, not knowing what was happening. I slurred and waved my hands frantically at Jeff as each muscle continued to contract tighter and tighter. Grasping his hand, I slowly slid to the tiled floor and waited for what seemed like forever for the contractions to stop. It was a night of terror. I sat on the toilet for the next few hours as my body seemed to want to clean out.

I WEPT.

I APOLOGIZED.

I WEPT SOME MORE.

This was not how I wanted our long-awaited vacation to turn out. This was anything but romantic, and it didn't remotely resemble a second honeymoon. I felt disappointed. I felt guilty. I felt terrified.

The morning sun cast a hopeful light on our day. We slid into our routine. I plastered on a smile as I drank my coffee. If I were being honest, I felt like a 120-pound bag of shit poured into a 50-pound sack. Every single muscle, including the ones I didn't know I had, were pained. I felt like I had just done a boot camp workout on back-to-back days. There wasn't any explanation that I could sum up. I had no idea what had happened, and neither did Jeff. All we could say was "What the fuck was that?"

We both kind of knew that something was really, really wrong. We both knew we had a few days left on our vacation and wanted to make the best of it.

I didn't drink at all that day. I lay around and didn't do much. I stayed out of the sun, ate small portions of food, and drank lots of bottled water. I even drank a well-known brand of electrolyte to ensure I was hydrated.

That night, I lay in bed and watched the ceiling fan, hoping its hum would lull me to sleep, but sleep evaded me. I noticed a numbing, tingling sensation in both feet that seemed to be creeping up each leg. I pulled back the sheets and used my cell phone's flashlight to examine my legs. I didn't notice anything and glanced at Jeff who was snoring in slumber, so I left him be and lay back down and drifted off.

More of the same routine followed the next day. I still wasn't feeling well. I was tired, achy, and my legs didn't feel normal. Each night, the tingling in my legs crept a bit higher until it made its way to my hips. I wondered what would happen if and when it hit my torso. Something in the back of my mind knew it wasn't going to be good, but I tried to remain positive.

On the night the tingling sensation reached my torso, I couldn't breathe. My breath was so short that I lifted my breasts to gain more room. I hobbled my way to the balcony door as I grabbed my robe. I wheezed as I plopped down onto the balcony chair with a thud. The scent of tropical flowers filled the air, and the cool night breeze felt good on my face. The tears streamed down my hot cheeks, as I knew I would have to wake Jeff. Something was seriously wrong.

When I entered the suite, the room filled with moonlight, but it no longer felt like paradise. And it no longer looked like it. The room seemed to spin as I slipped to the floor, cold tiles greeting my knees. Jeff, awake now, helped me back into bed. He placed a cool cloth on my head and rocked me as tears streamed down my face.

I wheezed the words, "I can't breathe, I can't breathe."

He handed me my inhaler. I took two quick puffs with hope that they would work to calm down both my mind and body. The inhaler failed to deliver. The breathing issues seemed to stem more from the muscles in my diaphragm than a tightness in my upper chest and throat. I watched the ceiling fan spin while Jeff held my hand and brushed away my tears. We both threw around the conversation of an ambulance and hospital. But we shook off the idea, as we were out of our element being out of country and having a medical crisis. We decided to wait it out.

By morning, I seemed a bit better. Coffee in hand, we walked slowly to the beach area under some beautiful palms. I kept up my water intake to stay hydrated. I looked at the beautiful turquoise sea and white sands framed by jungle-like foliage. My heart sank and tears streamed down my face. I wished it were a Canadian concrete jungle instead.

I felt horrible emotionally and physically and exhausted beyond anything I had ever felt before.

I stared off in the distance as Jeff approached with fresh cold bottled water. He smiled and took my hand to pull me up.

"Come stretch your legs." His smile was inviting as he pulled me along the white sugar beach. Guilt washed over me, and I plastered on a fake smile as I dragged my legs through the sand. We walked slowly and chatted about the sights. Not five minutes into our little walk, the breathing issues reappeared. I came to a halt, looking at him with doe-like glossy eyes.

"I'm really sick. I mean really, really sick. We need to go back."

It was a struggle to talk, to move, to think. My face was scarlet, and my heart was beating so fast it felt like it was going to thump out of my chest.

I collapsed into a lounger as Jeff ran full force to get medical help.

All I can say is that the medical facilities were archaic in the Dominican at that time. The ambulance ride was creepy, bumpy, and I felt like I had been teleported back in time. It was as if it was where all medical devices went to die after years of overuse in 1960. Things went from bad to worse when they demanded to hold our passports before delivering any form of medical assistance. The mini hospital was clean, yet *Twilight Zone* in nature. Everyone was speaking different languages, there were people crying, and the outdated equipment seemed straight from the set of *Dr. Kildare*. Having a health crisis out of country was not on any bucket list. But there I was living it—or dying from it.

I was hooked up to an EKG and monitor. It was done with suction cups, again very strange and frightening. A doctor emerged through the curtain. His English was accented and articulate. My blood pressure was through the roof and in the danger zone for a stroke. My heart rate showed tachycardia along with arrhythmias and A-Fib. I needed to go back to Canada immediately.

After all my out-of-country insurance was confirmed, they

released me, having done nothing except to say, "We have no idea what's wrong."

Back at the hotel, we researched an air ambulance out of the country. I spoke directly to the insurance company, as we had two days remaining in the Dominican. Air Vac would take a day to arrange, then a day to make it happen. They would Air Vac me to the US; I still wouldn't be in Canada. It would take the same length of time as waiting it out to get on our return flight to Canada. Decision made. We'd wait it out. I wanted to be back home. I wanted my own bed. I wanted to see my kids and tell them how much I loved them.

The two-day wait seemed like a month. I stayed in the hotel room in bed, and when I did get up, it was evident that I had mobility issues. I had jerky, wobbly leg movements. I couldn't remain up for long or the tachycardia would start up in full force. My face remained flushed. I was pooched.

Landing in Canada brought a sense of relief. I knew we would finally get some questions answered. I was rushed to a major Toronto hospital where the prognosis was . . . there was something not right. Could have been viral. Could have been allergic response. Could have been Guillain-Barre, but it was too late for testing. At that point, we headed for home, sweet home. All the "could have beens" overwhelmed me. I was exhausted mentally and physically. I had to take time off work to recover. I gave myself a week, then pushed myself to get back in the groove.

WAS I FEELING A BIT BETTER? THAT WAS DEBATABLE.

WAS I FEELING MYSELF? NO, I WAS NOT.

WAS I READY TO GO BACK TO WORK? NO.

WAS I IGNORING THE HEALTH FLAGS? YES, I WAS.

WAS I FEELING GUILTY ABOUT RUINING A VACATION? YES.

WAS I FEELING PRESSURE TO PERFORM AT WORK? YES.

WAS I FEELING EXTRA PRESSURE HOLDING A POSITION IN A MALE-DOMINATED FIELD? YES.

WAS I FEELING THE PRESSURE TO BE WIFE AND MOTHER? YES.

WAS I FEELING LIKE I NEEDED TO SLAP ON A FAKE HAPPY FACE? YES.

WAS I AWARE THAT THE ILLNESS WAS GOING TO HAUNT ME? NO, NOT IN A MILLION YEARS!

NOTE TO SELF

It's okay to ask for help. It's also more than okay to say NO!

Removing some of the hats you wear is not failure. It is not written anywhere that you have to wear them all 100 percent of the time.

It is okay to put your needs, your physical and mental health, first.

It's more than okay to rest, to heal, to take time for self-care. If you don't take the time to refuel, eventually you will run out of gas.

Your body is a temple, and you should worship it as it is the only vessel that will carry you through your journey!

Acorn

Be the strong oak you were born to be.
Let the storm take you,
Let it twist and shape you.
Let it rip away all that you are.

Branches will fall.
It will bend and almost break you.

The depth that you are planted in the soil
Is deep, deeper than all eyes can see.

The storm will pass,
You will emerge knowing
Birds with broken wings cannot fly.
Broken hearts break hearts that love.
A broken soul finds little joy.
Judgment stands with judgment.

Being burnt by a scorched tongue
Will only last as long as you let it.

Darkness always follows some,
Don't allow it to dim your shine.

Hope and tenacity are tattooed on your heart.

The depth of love and respect given out should be
equal to the depth of love and respect given back.

Let go of what no longer serves you,
Nurtures you.

Wondrous, positive growth is found in nurturing soil.
Plant your feet there, mighty Oak!

Give love freely, without judgments and expectations
as it is a reflection of you and says more about you than
it does about them.

TAKE A MOMENT FOR YOURSELF

Breathe, Pause, Reflect . . .

Have you had moments of crisis?

Were you able to let them go or have they haunted you?

A simple indicator as to whether you have healed, are still wounded, or are still healing is if you are triggered over the event or issue.

From my own perspective, time does not heal all wounds. Some wounds remain in the form of a scar. We have healed but are aware of the scar they have left. We acknowledge the scar, knowing we lived it in our past, but we are in the present. The only thing we can control about the wound is how we react to it in the present.

CHAPTER 8

THE BEGINNING OF THE END

The title of this chapter:

A. Is horribly tragic?

B. Hints at the final curtain call?

C. Is when the heroine loses it all?

D. All of the above.

Hindsight is 20/20, so I will just say this. In every end, there is also a beginning.

In 2011 I struggled physically, and to make matters worse,

I was bullied behind closed doors by a manager on the regular, and my only escape was out. Sadly, I felt like I needed to up my exit strategy plan as a wealth adviser. To do so, we needed to diversify. I decided that we needed to add real estate to our portfolio. We had planned a weekend away with our son Joshua and his fiancée Betsy in Niagara Falls. We would look at investment properties and have a wonderful weekend as well. Sounded like a win-win. Josh had just obtained his realtor's license, so it was a great opportunity to merge business and pleasure. I was looking forward to it. Niagara Falls had become a go-to for getaways for Jeff and me right from the beginning of our marriage. It was steeped with nostalgia and felt like a home away from home. It wasn't as iconic as the month-long cruise we did to Europe in 2008, but still, relaxation washed over me as soon as I entered the Hilton. The only disappointment was that my Hilton was booked out for a conference. But we booked rooms at another hotel overlooking the magnificent falls. They're a miracle, and one I never seem to tire of.

The weekend started off fine. I wasn't any more exhausted than what I had been enduring since 2006. There were good days and bad days. I was always trying to focus on the good more than the bad. We had viewings all lined up on that hot Saturday. By the time we came to the fourth viewing, my legs felt like lead.

"You okay, Mom?" Josh put his hand on my shoulder and looked at me with concerned eyes.

"I'm good, just tired." I gave him a half smile to reassure him I was good to go.

We entered the potential income property. The entrance had old twelve-by-twelve tiles. We stood shoulder to shoulder, trying to remove our shoes.

"Man, I am sweating," Josh said as he pulled at his crisp dress shirt.

I looked up at Jeff and could see he was sweating too. Small patches of perspiration marked where his golf shirt clung to his body.

"Why are you the only one not sweating?" Betsy asked, laughing as she dabbed her brow.

Shrugging my shoulders, I gave my usual response: "It's a gift; what can I say?" I forced a smile to make it seem like a joke. But I knew that it wasn't normal. It was one of those symptoms that didn't make sense to anyone, me included.

"I have heat intolerance; I don't know why I don't sweat. I just don't." Again, I smiled. My mind wandered back in time. I could hear a firm, authoritative voice stating, "Good God, Anne Marie, women do not sweat, they perspire."

"Mom, you okay? You look really flushed all of a sudden." Josh looked concerned.

"The house has mold." My response was abrupt and to the point.

"Come on. How do you know? We haven't even gotten past

the living room yet. Let's just give it a good look around; we're already here." Josh turned and pointed down the hallway to the bedrooms. "I'll lead the way."

We all followed in tow. He was right; it all looked good upstairs. But unfortunately, I was also right. I smelled mold right from the front door. Why no one else could smell it was beyond me. Again, I had the weird gift of hypersensitivity to odors.

I walked down the basement stairs and led them all to the back corner on the left side behind the washer. Lo and behold, the mold.

Pointing at the large patch of black, I jerked my shirt to cover my nose and mouth and made a quick exit while shaking my head. Nope, nada, ain't happening. "This house isn't for us."

We made our way back to the hotel. By the time I went to exit the car, I knew something felt off, really off. My breathing seemed a bit labored, and my legs felt worse than before. My heart rate seemed a bit too fast and abnormal with its pounding rhythm. Still, I insisted I just needed water and a bit of rest for twenty minutes, then I would be good to go. Honestly, I should have just stayed in the hotel, drank water, and crawled into bed. My need to please, my need to not be a party pooper and disappoint others got the better of me. I decided to push through how horrible I was feeling. I mean, after all, doctor after doctor and test after test had indicated there was nothing wrong. How could so many doctors be incorrect? Really, I mean what are the odds?

That night went from bad to worse. By the time we were seated at the Keg, I knew I was in real trouble. My face was still flushed, but I felt off, like I was functioning in a dream-like state.

I looked at Josh and Betsy across the table, my eyes filling with tears. "I need to go back to the hotel."

They seem surprised, perplexed.

"But you look fine, Mom. Your face isn't too flushed." Josh's eyes looked sad, disappointed, and concerned, all rolled into one.

Jeff ushered me to the elevator. At that point, I could barely walk. I started to collapse, and Jeff grabbed my arms to stop me from hitting the floor. I was taken by wheelchair to the hotel.

Once inside the room, my tears flowed, and my words were barely a whisper. "I'm so sorry. I ruined everything. Why is this happening? I'm so, so sorry." The guilt rushed over me, as did waves of adrenaline like I had experienced before.

"It's okay, babe. I know you can't help it. Don't worry, there will be other times, and we'll make it up then. But we will do your fave hotel the next time, okay?" He smiled as he kissed my forehead.

As he pulled his head from my forehead, he looked at me and took a slight step back. The reaction on his face said it all. He recognized in my eyes, as big as loonies, the zoned-out look I got. Then the confirmation of words that he knew on cue.

"I don't feel well. Oh, my God, Jeff, I don't feel well." I turned my head as I started to retch. My body and mind in unison becoming the calm before the storm.

Jeff coaxed me into the hotel bed and tried his best to get me under the covers. Then it started, the horrific attack. My teeth started chattering, the wild jerking of limbs, the slurring of words.

"Make it stop, make it sttop, mmakkke ittttt ssttopp . . ."

It was a violent attack. Time ticked for Jeff, but I lost all track of it. I surrendered to the uncontrollable attack as I had always done before, because honestly, it was too late to stop it, even if we knew how. All I could do was get through it.

I lay there in the king-sized bed, taking little space while looking at the falls. My eyes shifted over the skyline as the water and sky melted into one.

"Babe, hang in there. You've done this before, you're going to be fine, just breathe."

Jeff's voice reassured me all would be well.

Nodding slowly, I caught a glimpse of the lamp on behind him. Its dated and lackluster shade seemed out of place against the classic window-framed view.

"Babe, breathe, breathe. Maybe I should call 911, you're breathing too slow."

I shifted my focus back on Jeff's face, heard his words, and shook my head in a resounding no. We both knew it was useless. The ambulance had been called so many times, but nothing. Hospital visits, nothing. Specialist appointments, nothing. Just guesses and ruling out what it wasn't and accusations of "it's all in her head."

The attack seemed to go in waves as my muscles tried to ebb and flow with the contractions. Every tendon, ligament, and vein on my neck felt visible to the naked eye, bulging and stretching to their elasticized max. I tried to concentrate on something else as I listened to my teeth chattering rapidly, faster and faster like a flamenco dancer's castanets. No tears emerged from my eyes. It was as if they had cried too much in the past and felt the need to say enough is enough. My eyes blinked slowly, trying to focus on the wallpaper. Pale yellow mallows ran together in a mixture of muddy paints, blended like my painting pallet. The hues were washed from years of sunlight hitting the wall. Jeff's voice seemed quiet—or maybe farther away.

The view changed into a mist of white, and I felt as if I were floating. It was peaceful. There was no pain, no chattering of the teeth. My muscles were no longer contracted and contorted. I had never felt such a sense of peacefulness in my entire life. It felt as if I were floating in the mist, completely surrounded and levitated to an inner calm.

"Anne Marie, you have to go back. It's not your time." Her voice was kind and firm.

"Sweetheart, you've gotta go back." His voice was soft and convincing.

"It's not your time. Go back NOW!" Her voice grew louder and riveting.

"See you later, alligator. In a while, crocodile. GO, NOW!" His voice, playful, then insistent.

The mist was gone. I was transported back to the hotel room. Loud screaming buzzed into my eardrums. I saw Jeff's face, his eyes filled with panic. I felt his hand on my collar as he shook me.

"Babe, breathe, fucking breathe. Help me out, babe, breathe. Fuck! Fuck! Oh, God, breathe!"

I heard the wheeze as my chest rose to grasp air. His hands relaxed their grip as he pulled his trembling hands to his face. He emotionally melted in front of my eyes as I caught my breath.

"Where are they?" I scanned the room. "Where'd they go?"

"Babe, you fucking stopped breathing. This is fucked up. There is something seriously wrong. I don't care what they say. People just don't stop breathing." Jeff wiped his eyes and waited for my response.

"Where did they go?" I said, as if I didn't hear or even care about his alarming statement.

"Who? What . . . the hell are you talking about? Babe, did you hear me? You stopped breathing." He was exasperated. His face was drawn and exhausted from the shocking escalation of the attack.

"Nancy and Dad . . . where did they go?" I asked between tears.

"You know they've been dead for years. Do you know where you are? Do you know what year this is?" His voice sounded soft but concerned.

I nodded my head. "I know, I know. I gotta pee. Help me to the washroom."

It doesn't matter if you believe in life after death. It doesn't matter if you believe in heaven or hell. It doesn't even matter if you believe in reincarnation. Everyone is entitled to their own opinion and interpretation of their own thoughts on my near-death experience.

Was it a dream? I wasn't even asleep, so let's just call a spade a spade. That's a hard NO! It was as if my consciousness let go of my existing universe, allowing me to experience a state of consciousness where space and time do not hold us in this dimension. Rather than consciousness dying with the body when we pass, perhaps our body, our vessel, receives consciousness via frequency through matter. Some astrophysicists and physicists support the multiple universe, believing existing physical laws do not prohibit the possibility of parallel multiverse worlds. No matter how you look at it all, it's fascinating.

To me, the experience removed some level of anxiety that I had always held about death, about the unknown of it all. There's a fine line of having a normal curiosity about death. But I think when individuals become chronically ill or terminally ill, there is a higher level of consciousness about death. It began to cross my mind on a more frequent basis than say the average individual. In my reality, after that near-death experience, I feared not living life to the fullest more than I feared death.

NOTE TO SELF

Breathing is life itself. Your health should always be the number one priority. Finding and utilizing a practice of breath work is highly beneficial to your physical and mental well-being.

Self-care is crucial to healing. Make the time—and take the time—to heal.

TAKE A MOMENT FOR YOURSELF

Breathe, Pause, Reflect . . .

Have you ever pushed yourself due to your own expectations?

If so, why? What life lessons did you learn?

What would or could you do differently in the present?

Have you or do you know of anyone who has had a near-death experience?

When individuals become chronically ill, their thoughts on death sometimes change in narrative.
Has your own narrative about death changed?

If so, how and why has it changed?

We don't always have to have all the answers. Sometimes talking with a professional to work through difficult conversations, fears, and anxieties is the answer.

Afterlife

Your memory illuminates some of my dark passage of
time.

Like a glowing beacon urging me to go on to reach an
unknown shore.

Your voice echoing to demand my return to a life of
uncertainty.

Yet peaceful knowing you await my return in my final
physical moment.

CHAPTER 9

THE UNIVERSE THROWS BRICKS WHEN YOU DON'T LISTEN!

Life had gone back to somewhat normal after the huge episode in Niagara Falls. My career, our marriage, our children all continued to thrive; my health, not so much. I was fatigued and suffered weird and mysterious symptoms for which there didn't seem to be any explanation.

In 2012 my GI symptoms started to increase, as did a random rash. I was eating Gaviscon and Zantac like Tic Tacs. I was bloated and overweight and weighed down by endless pressure at work.

Frankly, it just wasn't the career pressure. The manager I had was an outright bully. And he didn't just bully me, he bullied all the females in my position. My complaints to head office fell on deaf ears. You would think in 2012 there would have been more repercussions. I assure you, he went unscathed. I cried in my car many a time as I watched other women leaving the company or being demoted from their position. I think what hurt the most was that my male coworkers knew and remained silent. I often wonder how they would feel if their daughters were treated in that manner.

The friends and family looking at my life did so with rose-colored glasses. They didn't see my struggles, nor did they hear about them. As 2012 began, I vowed it was going to be a great year. One filled with change. I was going to focus on my health plus building up our retirement portfolio. I was also going to build an exit plan from my book of business as a wealth adviser. I figured I had five years to build and implement my financial portfolio and exit strategy. I could do great things in those five years, but I needed to put the stepping-stones in place to reach those goals. And I needed to remain healthy to do so. After all, life is linear, is it not? I knew in my mind that it was not.

I also knew there was something very wrong with my health, even if the testing showed nothing. I didn't feel the same as I had in the past. Daily, I'd feel this inner vibration that would rise and peak and rise again. Just to be clear, this was a real sensation, as faint as it was; nonetheless, it was there in the pit of my stomach.

By February, after Valentine's, I'd focus on my new plan. Why wait? Well, we'd let the holiday parties pass, then get through New Year's and set our resolutions. I also needed to get past our wedding anniversary on January 2 and my birthday the week after. Figuring January would be partially a write-off anyway, I thought, *Shit, might as well wait it out until Valentine's Day is over*. So, I did.

The pasta, wine, cakes, and weekend espresso martinis were on the back burner. I was ready for the battle of the slight bulge and newfound energy that clean eating and exercise would bring. I went into it 100 percent. I booked a nutritionist, got a gym membership, and found a trainer. I was doctor-approved for these health and fitness goals. Sounded and looked great on paper, right?! No pain, no gain. Well, if there ever was a wake-up call, this was it. I was disciplined and regimented and motivated. Did I mention exhausted? Not the good kind like going for a run, finishing, and feeling like a million bucks afterward. Nope, more like feeling like major crap before doing anything. More like my body, mind, and soul wanted to lie down after a workout right there on the floor of the gym, crying, vomiting, and trying to breathe.

My trainer had said quite a few times during several sessions, "Are you okay? Maybe we should break" and "Why aren't you sweating? You know, I don't think I have ever seen someone work out so fierce and not sweat." She would shake her head in disbelief.

Another time, she asked, "Do you always go that color when you work out?"

Color? What color would that be? I mulled over her question in my mind as I turned to look full-on at myself in the mirrored fitness club wall. I tried to find my own reflection between the equipment and other health and body enthusiasts. Ah, there I was. Feeling lightheaded, I walked closer to get a better look, my trainer in tow.

"Holy shit, I look like a hot mess," I said, half-laughing and half-defeated.

My skin was mottled, bright red with a purple tinge. My lips looked dry and puffy.

I cocked my head sideways to change the angle of my reflection.

"Hey, do you see a pattern on my face?" I pointed to the mirror.

My trainer looked closer at my face.

"Not really a pattern, it's more discolored. But what the hell is going on with your hands? Why are they blueish? Furthermore, why aren't you sweating?" Her voice revealed a frightened level of concern.

I shrugged, as I had no answers, but it was the first time that someone other than in my immediate family had noticed that things didn't look normal with my strange and wild symptoms.

"I'm done for today," I said, shaking my head in disbelief and barely getting out the words. I knew the tears would soon follow. What the hell was wrong with me? The doctors said it's nothing. Why did I feel so physically horrible? Why was I so exhausted? What were all these strange symptoms that came and went? I felt like a walking example of shock and awe.

The next day, I could barely walk. My body was so pained. I was up retching all night. I had another "attack." I had to work from home that day and decided to start making a list of symptoms. I took a picture of my mottled skin.

I booked yet another doctor's appointment for the following day. This time, I went armed with notes and pictures on my phone. I had been brushed off by many a doctor because my symptoms hadn't seemed overly serious to any of them. Test results all came back negative, which is great, don't get me wrong. But when you feel like death warmed over, you would think that some form of test would show something.

The pictures and list of symptoms got me referred to a rheumatologist. I felt this was a positive thing. The day arrived, and I decided to just state my symptoms, show the pictures, and keep it brief and to the point. I knew the drill. I had already been to many a specialist and learned it was always a "hurry up and wait" and "keep it to the point" situation.

I left that day feeling heard. I felt I finally had someone in my corner. I left with my requisition to have more blood work done, which was a standard thing for me. Tests that were more specific to a specialist's area of expertise.

Stopping off at the lab on my way home, I sat in the parking lot of the clinic. I paused to take in the sparse trees in the lot, buds starting to emerge, their bases all freshly mulched. It wouldn't be long before new buds would pop in full bloom. It's amazing how trees lose their full spring and summer growth, working with all their might to let it all go in the fall. They pause, rest, then they do it again.

Maybe, just maybe, this was my spring. I felt physically and somewhat mentally beaten down a bit. Man, I was sick of being sick. Sighing, I walked slowly to the lab. My legs felt like they weighed a ton. I'd say I was dragging my legs if I didn't know better. Yes, maybe this was my spring. I needed to stay positive. Maybe I just needed more fresh air. Perhaps I should just try walking.

My test results from the rheumatologist came in quicker than I expected. I had very low levels of vitamin D. The recommendation was 50,000 UIs of vitamin D.

Sounded simple. But not so fast. Since 2006 my track record with taking any form of medication or supplements had been dicey. Actually, it was unpredictable and potentially dangerous. To be honest, it was more like if there was a possible side effect, I would get it, rash and all. The unpredictable part? Well, that became my new middle name when it came to my health. Since 2006 I had seemed to develop a huge list of allergies to medication, foods, chemicals, even the sun.

It took me all morning to convince myself that this was going to be just fine. Just had to pop that huge horse pill of vitamin D down, and I'd be good to go. A few deep breaths and a bottle of water and I seemed good, no biggie. Forty minutes later, I was lying naked, flat out on my bathroom floor, trying to decide which end I should aim at the toilet. My face was scarlet all on its own. My chest was all mottled in coloring. A small bead of cold sweat barely formed on the cupid's bow of my mouth. I felt like I was burning up. Crawling, I made my way to the shower and turned it on full blast with cold water. I sat there and time passed; time was irrelevant. My tears flowed, as did my fears. I felt this sense of slight panic that I had never experienced before, like a rush or dumping of adrenaline, rather than the usual wave.

Jeff came home at dinnertime that day on April 9, 2012, and found me in bed. My wet hair still wrapped up in the towel. My face still scarlet hours later. I wasn't hungry, just exhausted and frightened of the experience of the day.

I went to sleep early that evening while thinking that I just needed the day to be over, that the next day would be better.

I awoke at three to this horrible noise. My eyes flashed open, and I realized it was me, retching.

I jumped out of bed.

"Jeff, Jeff, wake up, wake up. Oh, my God. Oh, my God! I don't feel well. I don't feel well!" A sense of panic had set in. I felt this doom rush over me. My eyes showed my fear as he tried to coax me back into bed.

I dashed to the bathroom as the onslaught of retching restarted, lasting for about fifteen minutes. The force of it burst blood vessels in my cheeks. My abdominal muscles were contracting with such force that it caused me to pee all over the bathroom tiles. Then the retching stopped abruptly. My body and mind went quiet.

Back in bed, I felt doom wash over me. I knew too well that when the calm feeling set in, it was too late. The attack in all its wrath would begin within seconds.

My teeth started to chatter, my muscles all started to tighten, involuntarily contracting and jerking in different directions. My hands and wrists twisted and contorted inward until they couldn't bend anymore.

Stuttering, I looked at Jeff and pleaded, "Make it stop, make it stop, make it stop."

The final sentence came out inaudibly. My brain was still very aware of my surroundings, and I recognized my speech was so far gone that even I couldn't understand myself. Time passed and passed. I had had these attacks before. Every specialist I had gone to thus far couldn't figure it out. This time it was going on too long—ten minutes. Jeff made the decision to call 911. The EMS team and firetruck arrived quickly, catching the tail end of my attack. They noted the extremely elevated blood pressure and tachycardia. They also noted that my attacks were very "seizure/ convulsion-like."

The carpet had been pulled out from under my feet. I felt like I was in midair, watching the upheaval of everything in life I had created and balanced. The carefully constructed house of cards holding meticulously placed beautiful, marbled alleys piled neatly on top—into the air it all went, while I painfully and in slow motion tried to grasp it all and retain the balance to land on my feet. Each card toppled over; marbles went in different directions, all out of reach. In life, this time, the landing was a slippery slope; I toppled over the cliff's edge, dangerously, wildly flailing like a rag doll, hitting every tree branch on the way down. My resting place was face down, and the rest of my body dangled over the final cliff's edge. I clung to life by my fingernails. This time in life, I did not land on my feet.

That day was the beginning to the end of a chapter in my life.

I didn't know the day before was the last day . . .

that I would work as a wealth adviser.

The last day I would talk to my wonderful clients.

The last day I would socialize with my coworkers.

The last day I would hold down food.

The last day I would walk the dogs.

The last day I would socialize with friends at a restaurant.

The last day I would taste ice cream, pizza, solid foods, wine.

The last day I would prepare and enjoy a shared meal with family.

The last day I would be joyful for everything the holidays represent.

The last day Mom was Mom.

The last day my life partner, the love of my life, would have a whole Anne Marie.

The last day Anne Marie was Anne Marie.

The day before was the last day, and I didn't even know it. I just took the day as it was, not filled with gratitude, just a day, a plain old day like any other day—except it wasn't.

It was the last day of my first act, and I didn't even know it. In the blink of an eye, my entire world changed. The bell had rung for the second act. You know what they say: Once a bell rings, you can't un-ring it.

The ambulance ride that day seemed all too familiar. At that point in life, I was already on a first-name basis with several shifts of EMS staff.

The hospital emergency department and triage notated my blood pressure being extremely elevated and my tachycardia. Two IV bags and a couple of hours later, I was discharged when my vitals suddenly returned to normal.

My world came crashing down around me that day, and in reality, at that point in time, I had no idea that a life-altering shift had happened. The unplanned pivot had already happened in the blink of an eye.

NOTE TO SELF

When your body and mind softly whisper to take a break, to rest, heal, pause, or listen—honor yourself with the due respect it deserves.

TAKE A MOMENT FOR YOURSELF

Breathe, Pause, Reflect . . .

Have you had that moment in life when the "bell has rung?"

What feelings and emotions does it evoke?

What are some of the coping skills you can use to move forward?

If you lack coping skills and struggle, possibly reach out to a professional who can aid you with providing direction.

Fear & Truth

One should not try to conquer Fear
One should try to conquer acceptance of the Truth

Once you accept the Truth, the Truth will conquer the
Fear

CHAPTER 10

ACT II—THE FINAL CURTAIN CALL

Days rolled into weeks. Weeks rolled into months. My new life's routine was one from bed to bathroom, a bathroom that I crawled to even though it was but three steps away.

My symptoms were never ending, and the attacks were unforgiving, as they reminded me nightly in the wee hours of the morning. If nothing else, they were consistent, emerging to disrupt Jeff's sleep and my own between three and four, like clockwork.

LIKE A NIGHTMARE.

LIKE A SLEEPING GIANT WHO HAD BEEN POKED.

After four months, I had barely transitioned to the lower main level of the house. The onslaught of more specialists' appointments had started up again. I could barely drag myself out of bed.

I needed assistance to . . .

SHOWER.

DRESS.

EAT.

Get to the bathroom when the food wouldn't stay in.

I needed help to . . .

STAND.

WALK.

TIE MY SHOES.

GET TO APPOINTMENTS.

Some specialist appointments were in our area, some a far distance. At that point, both Jeff and I would have driven to the end of the earth to get answers, to get a diagnosis, to get treated, to get cured.

Honestly, by the ninth month, we had lost count of the number of specialists who had misdiagnosed me. And some had just offered opinions. Both left a bad taste in my mouth.

I had had more than my share of encounters with specialists.

From my perspective, they're a breed of their own. Spending years in university on their education before medical school, then even longer to specialize in their chosen field made them dedicated, intelligent, and focused. There were some, however, who had a level of arrogance and detachment and lack diplomacy, empathy, and consideration for a patient's perspective.

In the beginning, I held them in such a high regard, and I held onto this unrelenting grasp of hope. With every specialist appointment, there was a grain of hope. As long as there was hope, there was still a chance that life would return to normal.

Hope gets dashed many times when you are chronically ill. Sometimes it felt devastating.

We drove for four hours one way to see a well-regarded muscular specialist. The day was long, but we were both filled with hope and fear when we entered the medical facility.

We were greeted by the nursing staff who took notes and asked questions. I met with the doctor, and I insisted Jeff be present, as I wanted him to actually hear how some specialists talked to me. Was I being too sensitive, too critical of their lack of understanding and empathy?

The doctor entered, introduced himself, quickly read my file, then examined me. He announced matter-of-factly that if he couldn't figure out what was wrong with me, then no one could.

I stared at him in disbelief. Not in a challenging way, I just wondered which side of the line he was on—the side of confidence or arrogance? His next sentence solved that question.

"You're pretty much menopausal. So, either I will figure out what is wrong or it's all in your head. At the moment, I don't see anything wrong. You will have a fiber muscle test today, and we will have the results immediately." He departed abruptly, about as abrupt as his speech had been.

The test results were negative. His report to my family doctor was also negative. He stated that since there wasn't anything physically wrong with me, he thought my doctor should recommend mental health counsel.

I FELT APPALLED.

I FELT DISMISSED.

I FELT HOPELESS.

I FELT UNHEARD.

I FELT BLOODY PISSED OFF.

Not all specialists were like this, not even the majority. But there was just one too many who hinted that my being female, of a certain age and hormonal, was likely the issue.

Just to be clear, most individuals were leading very mentally and physically healthy lives prior to being taken down by a chronic illness. For the majority, it wasn't mental illness that caused the disease. It was the other way around. When an individual reached a point when they were finally classified as chronically ill, they were already physically and mentally beaten down. They had been through a war, battle after battle. Some had faced a lot of the battles on their own and tried to dredge through the illness wounded, feeling very alone, and isolated. Some have had to also then battle gaslighting, manipulation, and verbal and emotional abuse to add insult to injury. The order of progression generally was that the disease had taken away one's physical health, the prolonged disease became chronic, then the chronic and additional factors sometimes brought on mental health challenges.

Desperation seeps in when you are chronically ill as you watch the life you know slip away as you try to cling to hope that it will get better. Most individuals need a reason. I think the majority would ask the same questions.

WHY ME?

IN MY CASE, I ASKED MORE.

WHAT IS THE CAUSE?

WHAT IS THE DIAGNOSIS?

WHAT IS THE CURE?

WHEN IS IT GOING TO GET BETTER?

WHY HAVEN'T THE DOCTORS FIGURED IT OUT YET?

Being logical, I knew that desperation and wasting time on questions wasn't going to give me the answers I was looking for.

NOTE TO SELF

Listing all the questions (why, what, when) I had about my health, I realized that they needed to be whittled down to the singular most important question I needed answered.

How do I heal?

In reality, nothing else matters. Once healing starts, the rest will either fall away or come together, piece by piece.

Understanding your own narrative gives you a clear voice as to where your head is at, at that moment in time. Recognizing that a negative narrative will give negative results is imperative to healing. Implementing positive strategies and a positive narrative to that singular question of "how do I heal" is in reality one of the first steps in healing.

TAKE A MOMENT FOR YOURSELF

Breathe, Pause, Reflect . . .

Can you filter out all your burning questions and focus on a singular important question?

Can you then formulate a strategy so you move forward?

If not, who can you reach out to for support to help with your strategy to get the answer you need?

Do you agree with the statement that most individuals lead mentally functional lives prior to chronic illness, but that it's chronic illness and additional factors that usually lead to mental health challenges?

Healing the body requires a whole—mentally and physically—approach.

Do you have a starting point or a support team to address both aspects of healing?
If not, develop a plan to evenly balance your healing. If it seems overwhelming, take a step back and pause to consider finding a supporting health advocate who can assist you in creating your personal starting point.

CHAPTER 11

TIME TO TAKE THE BULL BY THE HORNS!

Various specialist appointments continued, closing the end of my first year of being chronically ill. Yes, I started to call myself that, mainly because my work status had changed as did anything that went along with my perks from my career. Short term ran into long term ran into chronically ill.

If anything, I am a resilient and determined woman. One with tenacity and a matter-of-fact attitude. I formally requested all my medical files. It raised eyebrows and cost me a minor bill to do so. I organized them in chronological order. I made a copy, then sent them via courier to a medical think tank in the US called "Best Doctors." It was one of the perks from my work benefits plan. There, a team of specialists would review the file. Then via group decision, they'd decide which area of medical practice was best suited to render a field of specialty. Once a field was closely matched, various specialists would formulate their letter of direction of diagnosis and treatment, if any.

Around the same time, I had decided to investigate my DNA. It was a public DNA company that also gave some results on personal health. I also decided to submit a second DNA sampling that leaned more into genealogy. I had always had a keen interest in both history and science, so the prospect of a new and interesting project seemed intriguing.

Why the hell not? I thought that maybe, just maybe, the personal health one would come back with something the doctors couldn't find. Did I want to find it, whatever it was? That was quite a loaded question. I have always been a believer of "be careful what you ask for."

Part of digging in and planting my feet firmly was the suggestion that my symptoms were all in my head. That I was this menopausal woman and therefore shouldn't be taken too seriously. I was made to feel at times like nothing more than a hot mess. In truth, this narrative is gaslighting. Simply put, it is a form of manipulation and a covert type of emotional abuse. The abuser creates a false narrative that makes the target question their reality and judgment.

I recognized that when I tried to summarize all my symptoms, it seemed like a lot. It seemed the symptoms came and went and came back again. They flared up. Then, as time progressed, a new symptom would emerge. Sometimes it was added to the flare-up; sometimes it would vanish. I had tried to describe my symptoms and condition in a short sentence, as I was frankly getting really sick of friends and family asking, "So, just exactly what is wrong with you? I mean, you look normal." This type of remark becomes common place when you live with an invisible disease.

The best I could sum it up was to say, "It's like I have hyperimmune response. It's like something turned the switch on and forgot to shut it off."

What exactly the switch was and where it was located in my body was to be determined at a later point in time. My body was hyper-responsive to everything: sound, light, sun, heat, smells, noise, touch. It was as if my body thought I was allergic to absolutely everything. When I say that, I mean full-blown rashes, swelling, hives, vomiting, diarrhea, breathing issues, GI symptoms, swallowing issues, neurological symptoms, mobility issues, brain fog, confusion, slurred speech, numbness, tingling, burning pain, abnormal bruising, dental issues, abnormal bleeding, visual issues. Oh, the list went on and on. The main reaction I tried to forget was the nightly attacks.

It was physically and mentally exhausting. It was also exhausting having to justify being chronically ill. No one should have to explain, justify, or defend themselves for having a chronic illness.

The Best Doctors' medical report arrived about eight weeks later. I held the large white bubble-wrapped package in my hands. Placing the package on my lap, I ran my fingers across the crinkle of plastic, looking at it as if it held all the answers of the unknown. My eyes welled with tears.

"Babe, aren't you going to open it? Isn't this what we have been waiting for?" Jeff seemed more eager than I was at that point.

"Yeah, yeah, give me a minute." My tone was already reflecting defeat. In the back of my mind, it was as if the seed of self-doubt had been planted by one too many specialists, making me feel that it could, in fact, be all in my head. After all, I was just like they said: a post-menopausal woman with zero tests that had produced any confirmed results. The post-menopausal condition had happened in my early forties due to an emergency hysterectomy. I had endometriosis and menorrhagia with nonstop bleeding. My ovaries probably resembled withered prunes at this point.

"Well, don't just stare at it, for God's sake. You open it up or I will." He'd always been a glass half full kinda guy, never the glass half empty.

"Think positive, babe. I've known you all my life. You and I know 100 percent that it is not in your head." He sheepishly handed me the scissors.

I jabbed in the package, my hands and wrists not having the dexterity to move my thumb and pincer finger to make a cutting motion. I gave up and Jeff took over the unveiling of the long-awaited report.

It was a professional presentation, and they also provided a USB drive with digital files. I flipped through the neatly constructed binder to make my way to the back pages.

"What the hell are you doing? Aren't you going to read it?" Jeff looked irritated to say the least.

"Later, I'll read it later. I just want to see if they have a diagnosis or prognosis or friggin something. It's not all in my head. I know it's not all in my head." The tears that welled up burst over the rims of my eyes, down my cheeks, and onto the pages of the medical report. I blotted my eyes while Jeff blotted the tears from the page.

Deep breath, Anne Marie, you can do this. My internal narrative was on point, even if in that moment I felt I was not. *Just breathe—inhale, exhale, inhale, exhale—and turn the bloody page!*

Validation is half the battle!

There it was at the top of the page: Probable diagnosis—Mast Cell Activation Disorder/Syndrome (MCAD or MCAS).

There was a list of recommendations and notations, including one for a Toronto immunologist who had vast knowledge of the disorder and was cc'd on my file. Frankly, I was not surprised by the diagnosis, as I had previously read medical articles and reports on the disorder. I was mildly vindicated. Jeff seemed excited and proclaimed victory before he understood what the diagnosis even meant. I wasn't quite ready to do a victory dance. I already knew there wasn't a clear-cut cure, only treatment and management. I forwarded the information to my family doctor.

As we headed off to bed that night, there was more hope than the day before. Jeff seemed so upbeat. He was adamant that I was going to be cured. He refused to even let me utter the full sentence containing words of "no cure," cutting me off abruptly.

"Don't you even say it. Just don't. I don't want to hear you say that again. You don't know. The doctors don't know shit. Some of them said it was all in your head. So don't say there is no cure. I don't want to hear it. Not tonight, not ever. The doctors know jack shit. They can't figure out shit about you. They can't figure shit out about my dad. I don't want to hear anymore tonight. I need to get some sleep. Let's go to bed, okay?" Jeff's face looked tired and pained.

It was the first time but not the last that his frustration, fears, and anger about the uncontrolled life's turn of events would be aired.

"Okay, babe. Let's head to bed. Do you mind if I sit up and read for a bit?" I already knew that answer: he wouldn't care. Honestly, the man had always been able to fall asleep with the lights on. Even if a train sped through the bedroom, he would have just rolled over and continued snoring.

MAST CELL ACTIVATION DISORDER/ SYNDROME

It's a condition when the body releases mast cells and other inappropriate amounts of chemicals. The condition causes an inappropriate systemic response. Symptoms are widespread and vary: hives, rashes, breathing issues, GI issues, anaphylactic reactions.

Sitting up in bed, I shifted toward the night table lamp in a desperate attempt to read the report; my eyes were tired but not in a sleepy way. It was as if the muscles in my eyes were fatigued, which sometimes made it impossible to read.

Scanning the pages, one line caught my eye. The use of language in the usual clinical format didn't faze me. What caught my attention was the use of primary and secondary conditions. The Best Doctors' specialist indicated that Mast Cell Activation syndrome was secondary, meaning there was an unknown primary condition. He also indicated that chances were that I had more than one secondary condition from the primary. Honestly, it was late, and maybe I wasn't reading it correctly. Maybe I just had too much brain fog to take it all in. I didn't understand the sentence. Did that mean we were looking for something else as well as mast cell activation syndrome? What the hell did that mean? My brain couldn't think anymore. My body ached. I looked at my phone; it was 1 a.m. What were the chances that I would get woken at 3 a.m. with an attack? I am not a betting woman, but I would place a cool million on that bet. Making my way slowly to the ensuite for my last pee of the night, I questioned it all.

I'd had so many gaslighting me that I was on the verge of throwing in the towel and just saying back to a few of those doctors and people, "You're right, all that is wrong with me is made up in my head."

It all went from the gaslighting thoughts ingrained in my head to a complexity of more than one condition. WTF?!

Washing my hands, I glanced in the mirror. I barely recognized myself. My cheeks were hollowed out; I had deep, dark circles under my eyes. My eyes' reflection was dull as if the life had been sucked out of me. My hair had gone white and silver and was patchy in spots, coming out in handfuls at times. I had marks on my face from the allergic blisters, made worse by my uncontrollable urge to pick at them. Leaning in toward my reflection as I ran my hands through my hair, a slight smile crossed my lips. The day was and should be considered a victory. Proof it was not in my head. Granted, in this moment, I looked like a hot mess.

That night, I would have lost that bet, hence why I am not a betting woman. The attack didn't come at 3 a.m., it came at 4:30 a.m. FML! I bet there isn't a chronically ill person out there who hasn't screamed "fuck my life!" at some point. Maybe, just maybe, I will take that bet. I hear you. I see you. I feel every ounce of your anger and frustration. I feel the salt that's rubbed into the wound when people we trust and respect use gaslighting as a response to and cause for our chronic illness.

NOTE TO SELF

Don't ever allow someone, anyone, to diminish your thoughts, words, feelings. Stay strong in your goal, the one of healing. Be the strong health advocate you need. If you feel you can't provide yourself the necessary advocacy, find someone you can lean on who has shown you in your past that they are capable, reliant, and strong and that they have your best interests at heart.

TAKE A MOMENT FOR YOURSELF

Breathe, Pause, Reflect . . .

Have you experienced gaslighting? It's a form of manipulation that is used to diminish someone's sanity.

The moment anyone starts to diminish your thoughts, feelings, or emotions, it is gaslighting.

You deserve to have your thoughts, feelings, and emotions validated. It's called RESPECT!

Holding your own and keeping integrity is difficult at the best of times, and it's even more difficult when you are chronically ill.

When met with gaslighting or highly confrontational individuals, try to remove the emotion or defuse it by simply replying with "I am not sure if the direction of this conversation is productive."

Or "Perhaps we can pause this direction of conversation."

You are so worthy of respect!

Where Are You!

I was there when your world fell apart, numerous times, I might add.

I was there to hold your hand, talk you through the battles.

I was there, a soft spot for you, both hands open to brace your fall.

I was there to listen, hear your side, your thoughts, validate your feelings, as you wore the label "black sheep."

I was there to show unconditional love.

I was there to base the truths by your mouth and not the mouths of others.

I was there with respect, truths, honesty, and love.

Now the tables are turned. Where are you?

CHAPTER 12

DISH IT OUT—I'M DISHING IT BACK!

Waiting for a referral for the immunologist appointment seemed to take forever. The system was backlogged. I had already been submitted to a different specialist months prior and still had not heard back.

I seemed to be in a constant state of flares that would just not settle down. It was a very rough time. I had reached the point that I was having hyper-response reactions to everything, including water to drink and bathe in, plus my own tears, which now caused hives.

Okay, rough is a huge understatement. It was horrific! The longest I went without eating was over thirty days. I weighed in at eighty-seven pounds soaking wet. I was sleep-deprived, starving, and mentally beaten down beyond anything I had ever experienced.

The immunologist and dermatologist appointments could not arrive fast enough.

Here comes that tag line again: "Be careful what you ask for." The appointment dates were confirmed two days apart. It would be a stressful week, more physically than anything. I knew one appointment was exhausting and a ride could be arranged, but two pretty much back-to-back? I knew I would pay for it in the end, health wise.

Nevertheless, I got it done. The mast cell appointment was successful all around. I had a classic case and was told it would take a hit-or-miss approach to figure out what medication I could tolerate and what I could not. Also, it would take time to baby the medications in. "It's not a cure. All we can do is manage it." Even the specialist looked tired and sad from saying that line one too many times to patients.

The surprise about the visit was his look of knowing when he read the report. The doctor on the report was known to him. He, too, agreed that MCAD was secondary and not the primary cause. It was the first time a feeding tube was mentioned. If my symptoms didn't improve with medications, we might have to move in that direction. The immunologist made note that a lot of my symptoms didn't fall into MCAD, but instead fell into the category of postural orthostatic tachycardia (POTS).

Come again on that one? Postural orthostatic tachycardia was another rare disease. But are they truly "rare," or are they perhaps more so misdiagnosed, undiagnosed, delayed in diagnosis? By support group member numbers in numerous groups, I would beg to differ about the rarity statement. There was also a chance I had Ehlers-Danlos syndrome (EDS), which would be considered more rare.

The long day in Toronto left me with prescriptions, hope, and a referral to two other doctors.

I made it in one piece to my second specialist appointment that week. Too weak to walk, I needed to be taken into the hospital by wheelchair. My closest friend of twenty-three years had semiretired and was spending winters down south. She'd been gone quite a bit over the last few years, readying her place in the Bahamas. But she was here at the right time and offered to take me. Patty hadn't seen me since I had become ill. She was busy preparing the island home and catching up with business while I was just trying to survive. The shock on her face when she laid eyes on me said it all. She tried to not show it, she really did, but the vast difference to what I had been before was striking. That day was also a pivotal point for us as friends. It was the beginning of a distancing between us by country and by circumstance. She was going through the horrific battle of cancer with her beloved sister Brenda.

Patty had commented a number of times after this turning point:

"I just can't do this." Tears filled her eyes. Her hands waved in the air.

"Do what, Patty?" My linear mind tried to follow her comment, but I didn't understand what "this" meant.

"This," she said in a whisper, pointing at me and her. "It's a lot, you know." Her words were barely audible.

The brief time we spent together resonated with her in an overwhelming way. I didn't understand it then, but now I think it must have been difficult for her to watch her closest friend wither away from the unknown while also watching her sister battle terminal cancer and a stroke. Patty eventually lost her sister to cancer, and she just couldn't lose someone again. She just couldn't watch helplessly as someone she loved lost their battle. I felt abandoned by her after that point in time. I was angry at her lack of support. I would have been there for her. I didn't hold back the fact I was angry. I also didn't recognize at that time that she really, really couldn't do "this" again.

I was also angry about the chronic illness and the shitty cards I had been dealt and was still being dealt. We reached an unspoken understanding at that point in our friendship. Later, though, I spoke my truth about how I felt, and she did as well. We each said "sorry" and moved on with life. The change in both our lives distanced in many ways. I can only speak for myself, but sometimes you need space to heal. Sometimes you need space for growth as individuals.

We hung in there as very close friends, eventually finding our way back to each other. Patty is still my "ride or die," one of my closest friends. We cheer for each other, hug it out, and cry it out. We clap for and support one another. Many, many years ago, Patty's beautiful mother, Phyllis, took me aside and said, "There will be times in the future when you will want to let Patty's hand go, or she will want to push you away as her heart just can't take on the world. Promise me you will always stay connected, even if it's the tiniest of ribbons, long and strong enough that you can reel her back in. You are both cut from the same cloth: strong, independent, driven, un-needy women. One day, you're both going to figure out that you need each other more than either of you realize."

At the second specialist appointment of the week, Patty was there, front and center, driving me downtown and wheeling me into the hospital. I had become too weak to walk. I had fought the assisted mobility aspect of life; my mind didn't want to go there. On that day, I didn't fight it. I knew that I'd never make it out of the underground parking lot alone, never mind make it to the appointment through the vast hospital maze of halls and elevators.

I was closing in on two years of being chronically ill. I seemed desensitized to some things in life and overly sensitive to other things. That statement was accurate for both my body and mindset. Survival is one thing, but actually living is completely different. I felt like I was stuck in survival mode. "Flight or fight" described it more accurately.

One of the good aspects (or possibly bad, depending on how you view it) was that I had become somewhat desensitized to arrogant comments or opinions. Trying to cope, I coupled them with humor, usually sarcasm. Either I was getting bitchier, or my mind was functioning better because I usually had quick and witty responses to dish out when needed.

My second appointment of the week was at one of the teaching hospitals. I am in favor of teaching hospitals and applaud their hands-on approach to patient care; however, as sick as I was, I wasn't about to be the quiet test study for them.

The doctor came into the examination room, followed by four interns who were probably filled with either curious wonderment or boredom.

"Well, ladies and gentlemen, we have a bit of a zebra," the doctor said, addressing the interns, waving the chart in my direction.

After introducing himself, he started off by giving an overview of my symptoms and medical history. The stage was clearly his, and he felt more directed to the interns than me. Honestly, I felt like a guinea pig on display. He talked to them as if I wasn't even in the room. I sat ever so quietly, taking in the interns' faces as the specialist kept his eyes down to read the details on my chart. The interns stood silently with nothing more than a slight shift in body weight. At times, they didn't seem to know where to keep their gaze. They were taking in the details in a relatively detached manner.

The specialist continued to read the words and symptoms I had heard too many times over. His monotone voice made it easy to drift to other thoughts as I surveyed the faces of the interns.

All that schooling and now specializing in dermatology—why? I'm not knocking the field. My question was more, if you choose to specialize, wouldn't one think it would be a passion or a field that intrigued you? But right then, no one in the room seemed passionate or intrigued. I was hoping I misjudged the specialist's audience. My mind wandered off while my eyes looked them up and down; I tried to assess if any words coming out of the specialist's mouth would pique their interest.

I suddenly realized that all eyes were on me.

"Mrs. Key Well, that question was directed toward you?" The specialist's voice was firm and slightly annoyed.

Feeling a bit startled and out of place, the best response I could summon up was a quick question back.

"I'm sorry, can you repeat the question please?" My voice sounded clinical as if I were on a game show and was about to answer the final round of questions for the big money.

"Your history indicates that you began birth control pills at the age of fifteen. There is no indication of brand of birth control pill. What was the brand?"

"The brand? You want to know the brand of birth control I used when I was fifteen?" I said, questioning why the hell that would make a difference now.

"Yes, Mrs. Key Well. What was the brand?"

"Please, call me Anne Marie. Honestly, I can't remember the brand. That was like thirty-five years ago."

"Come now. It was your first birth control pill; surely you can remember the brand." The specialist shook his head slightly in disappointment and rolled his eyes in exasperation.

Rather than feeling like some idiot who failed to answer what to him seemed like a simple question, I summoned up a sarcastic response.

"Tell me, Doctor, can you remember one of your first sexual encounters? What was the brand of condom you used? I mean, I am guessing it was roughly thirty-five years ago as well. What brand was the condom?" I smirked at him as his face turned beet red.

The interns' serious demeanor dissipated into rounds of giggles. The more they tried to control it, the worse it got. Someone even snorted in laughter.

The specialist had lost control of the stage, lost his audience.

"Out, everyone out!" He pointed the interns toward the door. "You stay right here," he said, pointing at me.

I sat there on the examination table, trying not to crinkle the white paper. It's not that I cared about the paper, I just didn't want to make any noise so I could hear them in the hall, just outside the door. However, all I could hear were muffled voices. Well, that just wasn't going to cut it. I wanted to hear what was being said, as it was more entertaining than anything else. I just needed to get closer to the door. Quietly, I placed my hands on the crisp paper and pressed down so it held my weight as I edged myself off the table. I learned there was no quiet way of doing this. My one leg dangled, the toe of my Converse shoe barely touching the step up. My gown edged up in the process, showing my thigh as I stretched my short legs to the max.

Just then the door flung open.

"Now, where were we?" The doctor looked slightly agitated.

My face must have shown my surprise, and in my awkward stance, there was nothing to do but smile, so I gave them my best "kid with their hand caught in the cookie jar" smile I could muster up. I must have looked exactly that because the interns started to giggle yet again. The specialist was pissed. He did his best to grab back control of the room. Me, I didn't give a shit. I just wanted the appointment over at that point.

"Enough," he said, giving a glare of death toward the interns. "Moving on, shall we?"

I left the appointment that day with new medical vocabulary and a better understanding of some of my symptoms, as well as with an additional diagnosis: Chronic urticaria with high probability of autoimmune-related with visible dermatographic urticaria.

I also left feeling slightly vindicated with the confirmation of my symptoms and slightly victorious about my successful round of sarcasm.

Patty wheeled me to the underground parking lot. I gave her the entire recap of the appointment. By the time we had our seatbelts buckled up, we were laughing so hard that we were both in tears. I thanked her over and over for that day's support.

NOTE TO SELF

Take up space!

Step into the light; you deserve to be seen.

Doing the best you can is, in fact, good enough!

Honor yourself when disrespect is dished out.

Call it out, lay it all out there, or walk away!

TAKE A MOMENT FOR YOURSELF

Breathe, Pause, Reflect . . .

Laughter is like medicine.

Have you had moments in life when you laughed so hard you cried? Laughed so hard you snorted, coughed, and almost peed yourself?

If you can't remember the last time you had that type of deep laughter, then it's overdue.

Part of self-care is allowing yourself to lose yourself to something positive that stimulates positive emotions. Try scheduling time to take in a few feel-good, laugh-your-head-off kind of movies. An actor's best wish is to transport you to where they are so they can entertain you and make you laugh, even for a brief period of time. Laughter is medicine! Take the medicine.

Shine!

Pause,
Be Still,
Breathe,
Soul Search,
Stay Authentic,
Follow Your Heart,
Step into the light and embrace your Shine!

CHAPTER 13

WHAT POKES THE MONSTER?

As time passed, each day seemed like the last. The doctors' appointments seemed endless. Blood work was futile. I was two years into this mystery illness, and my life had reached both a breaking point and validation, which in itself was bittersweet. I finally had a diagnosis: mast cell activation, hyper-POTS, and EDS. I was told there wasn't any point of doing more testing. There wasn't any point of looking into anything else. There just wasn't any point at all. "It is what it is," they said.

I didn't buy it. Was I pissed off? Yes! Did I think I was smarter than they were? That they were wrong and I was right? No, I didn't feel that way entirely. Not smarter, anyway. I just had this aching feeling that they were wrong with some of their diagnosis in relation to EDS. I also felt that there was a chance I could heal, that I would get better. Maybe that was just denial of both my journey and the illness itself. It's often easy to lump health cases into a category. It makes it easier for specialists and therefore there's no need to continue to look further. They diagnose, then move on. The pushback to the family doctor to maintain and manage the patient is real.

At the two-year mark, I no longer remembered what it was like to not have a day without pain. I didn't know what it was like to not feel sick. It was endless and unrelenting. The emotional toll it took to remain sane and the strength it took to slap on a fake happy face was absolutely draining.

I was blindsided by the fact that some family and friends lacked empathy and understanding. They almost bullied me to death. I often thought about ending it all because of both the physical pain and the emotional pain of the bullying, shaming, and verbal abuse that was unleashed on me.

One thing I've learned about all this is that any turmoil and drama present in a relationship before an illness arises only escalates afterward. Sadly, I can still hear their words in my head. I think the one that stung the most was: "Go ahead, Anne Marie, use that sick card."

I'm sure you'll agree that there is a huge difference in someone hurting your feelings unintentionally and inflicting words upon you with the intent to wound.

One particular day was especially bad. You know, the kind of day when you are so mentally and physically exhausted to your soul that you can't even talk about how your day was. You can't be bothered to express to someone at the end of it how horrific it was. All you can say is that you just need the day over so you can hopefully start fresh the next morning. It was a day from a new level of hell that had followed three nights and days of hell before it. I was paying for having specialist appointments back-to-back. I wasn't just flaring up, I was on fire. My body and mind were depleted from the endless retching, hives, and horrific attacks.

"For God's sake, please someone, anyone, explain to me what these attacks are. I can't take it. I just can't do it anymore. I'm done. Seriously, I'm done!"

The new antihistamines were hard to get in and keep in. It was day four of no sleep, no food, and a scarlet-red face that was burning up. I was alone in the house, except for my Yorkies. My sweet Abby never left my side. She was a godsend. She knew me before and during my illness. My sweet, sweet girl never changed her level of devotion. She comforted me and warned me before each attack started. How she knew is beyond me, but she knew. Less than a minute before each attack, she would snuggle up and place her chin on my hand and just look at me as if to say, "I'm here, Mom. It's coming. I can feel it. I can smell it. I love you, Mom." She was my special girl. My fur baby, my sweet Abigail.

I lay there on my ensuite bathroom floor, my face pressed to the tiles to cool my burning cheeks. My only movement was to turn my cheek to find a cooler tile. Emotions welled up inside me. I wailed. I screamed. I begged God, the God I had detested when I lost Jenna. I wailed some more. I screamed to the universe with hatred. "Why the fuck didn't you just kill me with the first attack? Why do I have to suffer like this?"

I had passed the relieved point of feeling happy that I had survived and had reached the point in chronic illness where I realized this relentless, unforgiving anguish was my reality—the part of chronic illness when you realize you are alive, but you are not living.

THE PART WHEN YOU REALIZE EVERY DAY IS A STRUGGLE.

THE PART WHEN YOU REALIZE THAT THIS SHIT ISN'T GOING AWAY.

THE PART WHEN YOU FEEL HOPELESS.

THE PART WHEN YOU FEEL YOU WOULD HAVE BEEN BETTER OFF DEAD.

THE PART WHEN YOU FEEL YOU JUST CAN'T TAKE IT ANYMORE.

"I am SO fucking done! Do you hear me? I'm done!"

My tears caused my face to erupt into migrating hives. I was inconsolable—I had deep, gut-wrenching wails as if the world was ending. I moved from begging God to bargaining with God. I felt borderline hysterical as I lay there ugly crying, tears and snot running down my nose like a child. It lasted for about three hours until complete and utter exhaustion closed in. Until tears no longer fell from dehydration. I curled into the fetal position, half naked on the bathroom floor, not giving a fuck about myself anymore.

The house was silent as I looked sadly at my beautiful Abby who never left the threshold of the bathroom door. She raised her chin off the carpet, just enough to meet my level of sight, waiting for me to talk to her, to let her know I was okay.

"I'm okay, Abby. Mommy will get up in a minute."

She lowered her head back down and waited for me, not moving from her on-guard position.

My mind wandered as I lay there quietly, still trying to cool my cheeks and catch my breath. Then I had an aha moment. Not a life-changing moment, but one more of growth, I would say.

Being a vivacious reader, I suddenly remembered a book from 2006. I couldn't wait to read it when it came out. I had snatched up a copy as soon as it was available in February that year. The title involved a lot of praying, loving, and eating. At the time, as much as I tried, I just couldn't get into the book. I know, I'm probably one of the few who felt that way because it was a major hit. It wasn't like I didn't give the book a few goes. I really did give it an honest effort. The main issue I had with the book was its main character, especially when she had a meltdown on her bathroom floor. I stopped reading then and protested out loud at her.

"Oh, for fuck's sake, get your ass off that bathroom floor and change something about your life. Grow some bloody balls, will you?"

And so, I put the book down in protest. I just didn't get the main female character; I just couldn't relate to her level of desperation.

I finally got it. I finally felt the level of desperation the writer was trying to portray. I suddenly not only felt for the main character, but I also felt such empathy toward the author. As a writer, you dig into and try to capture a level of emotion, but this writing had to have come from a level of perception only by experience. Now, not only did I have empathy, but I also had compassion.

My aha moment of growth was coming to the realization that a person's level of perception can be truly and deeply based on their own experiences. As hard as anyone tries to bring understanding and empathy, it can only go so far as to their experiences in life. Compassion, however, is something that all individuals should be capable of. I vowed then to retrieve the bestseller from my bookshelf, blow the dust off it, and give it another try.

I read it in two days, tissues in hand. I thought it was one of the best books I had read. I could not put it down. Growth happens on its own schedule. In my meltdown moment on my bathroom floor, I had a breakthrough on many levels. It was a turning point, a catalyst to a degree.

I got off the bathroom floor that day, partially because of my newfound level of perception, and partially because there were dust bunnies in the corners of the bathroom. I remember thinking that I couldn't die and leave behind a dirty bathroom. My mom brain also kicked in for my fur baby, thinking she probably had to pee and needed food and water. So, I dragged myself up first to my hands and knees. Then I gripped the vanity sink. I wiped the snot and tears away. I washed my face, then took a deep breath while looking at my unfamiliar reflection and announced, "This shit is not going to win! This disease is not—I repeat NOT—going to rule my life! I don't care what the doctors say. I don't believe I should just accept this is as good as it gets! Screw that! Screw them!"

My fight-mode warrior was kicking in, and I summoned up the strength to battle on. Damn, I had missed her.

NOTE TO SELF

This is but a moment in time. Moments pass; this will also pass.

Chronic illness ebbs and flows. Take in the spans of time when the monster is sleeping. If the monster gets poked and reminds you it is still there, acknowledge it and give it what it needs so it can go back to sleep.

Take care of yourself.

Sleep, keep hydrated. Implement positive daily practices, meditations, breath work.

Your attitude matters. You matter!

Saying "No, I can't do this today" is a strength, not a weakness. Keep strong, if only in mind.

Start a positivity journal!

TAKE A MOMENT FOR YOURSELF

Breathe, Pause, Reflect . . .

Promoting self-care is feeding your mind with positive narrative, which promotes calm, peace, and joy. And it can uplift you.

Creating a positivity journal and adding it to your healing journey routine is a strong positive behavior. It is nurturing to both mind and soul.

Can you dedicate three minutes per day to promote self-care?

If you feel it's too much to dedicate, I ask you this: If it was your loved one who needed you to give them three minutes of your time to nurture their mind and soul, would you gladly give it to them? If yes, then recognize that you, too, are worth the time for self-care.

Today Is Not a Good Day

Today is not a good day for me.
Today is a day I wallow in self-pity, anger, and fear.

Today is not a good day for me.
Today is a day the emotion is so intense it flows down my cheeks.

Today is not a good day for me.
Today is a day the last attack is etched in my mind.

Today is not a good day for me.
Today is a day my fears were exposed as all hope and courage have been ripped away.

Today is not a good day for me.
Today I am like a starving dog, beaten each time it has been fed.

Today is not a good day for me.
Today I fear the hand that feeds me.

Today is not a good day for me.
Today I will painfully hold on as I wait for tomorrow, because my story isn't over yet.

CHAPTER 14

VINDICATION, ROUND TWO

Approximately eight months later, I had my appointments with the cardiologist for postural tachycardia syndrome and with the dermatologist for Ehlers-Danlos syndrome.

As with all my other specialist appointments, I read up on the suspected diagnosis so I would have a clear understanding of the disease or syndrome. It also prepared me to ready questions and feel prepared for how they would relate to my symptoms. These appointments were no different.

The dermatologist appointment was first up, and it was quick.

There was only one intern to deal with my complete medical history. I didn't fit the mold of EDS. As a child, I didn't have any problems with my joints or issues of constant dislocations or unusual bruising or healing issues. Yes, GI issues from time to time, but overall, it just didn't fit. I felt in my heart that they were looking for the wrong link to my chronic illness. My gut told me that, as did my medical history when I broke it all down. I was sure that the chronic illness started as viral or perhaps bacterial, and I truly believed as I walked out of the hospital that day that the diagnosis of EDS was wrong.

I felt that several teams of doctors wanted to connect the dots into this triangle of MCAD, EDS, and POTS. But I didn't quite fit that mold. I had to wait until 2020 to confirm that I was right. I had a two-year wait with a renowned clinic for EDS. A team of doctors who specialize in only it finally confirmed 100 percent that I did NOT have EDS. Did I have hypermobility issues? Yes, but those issues didn't really become problematic until I was chronically ill.

A few weeks later, the POTS appointment was arranged. The cardiologist was a three-hour drive away, one way. I was tired by the time I got there, but it worked out well that Jeff could take me to this appointment.

The waiting room was packed. "Hurry up and wait" seemed to be the theme. No one's fault. It was just the course of the day. I was ushered in to have an EKG. Not long after, the cardiologist came out and the appointment proceeded. It was nothing out of the ordinary. The usual medical history. At the time, the specialist was looking at the fact I had a confirmed diagnosis of MCAD and also EDS. It didn't change the diagnosis of POTS, but in moving forward for treatments in the future, my guess was that it would. It didn't take long for the cardiologist to confirm the POTS diagnosis. The only missing piece was which type of dysautonomia (autonomic nervous system disorder) I had. Some professionals in 2021 would rather the subtypes of dysautonomia not exist; however, I personally feel it is important to distinguish each, as the symptoms and treatments are different.

A tilt table test a few months later confirmed I had a substantially raised level of norepinephrine in my blood during the test and blood draw. That marker gave the confirmed diagnosis of hyper-POTS. I left that day feeling validated. There was an actual blood test that showed an abnormal result.

If you have ever been chronically ill, yet zero tests prove that you are in fact chronically ill, you feel bloody vindicated when there's finally medical proof. But it's a bittersweet kind of feeling. You want to yell at the top of your lungs:

"I told you there was something wrong."

"I told you I was sick."

"I told you it wasn't in my head."

"I told you, damn it! I told you so!"

I left the cardiologist that day feeling hopeful. I also left holding two prescriptions without knowing how I was ever going to get them in. I felt a sense of *okay, what do I do now?*

There were a lot of specialists who I'd been to that like to make the diagnosis, give a recommendation of medication, but then do not manage the patient. This cardiologist was one of those, making it clear the moment the diagnosis was made. There was no confusion in the words:

"I do not manage you as a patient. I diagnose. I recommend medication. Your family doctor manages."

So, where did this all leave me at that point in time? I had a diagnosis of mast cell activation, EDS, and dysautonomia in the form of hyper-POTS with no management team in place.

WTF?!

A diagnosis is a label, but management is action. Those who are chronically ill need management to successfully give them a better quality of life. No management equals falling through the cracks of a medical system.

Seriously, are you feeling me here?

A diagnosis without the proper management team working together for the best outcome is a shit show. Talk about a sheet hanging on a clothesline during a tornado and hoping the sheet survives!

NOTE TO SELF

Make notes. Write a journal. Write a book. Write it all. Put it all out there. To hell with others who do not understand your calling; they were not meant to understand it. My calling is for me to understand that this was not a conference call.

Be the biggest and strongest health advocate you can be. Be the badass warrior for your inner child and nurture and care for yourself. You will heal. This is bigger than you. You will find a way to rise, then you will help others to rise. You are a warrior!

TAKE A MOMENT FOR YOURSELF

Breathe, Pause, Reflect . . .

Have you ever been scarred by life?

Did it leave a wound?

Is it a wound that has healed?

Can you talk about it without crying? If you can be reminded of your "life before" without anger, heartache, or depression, that is a good indicator that it has healed.

If you find you are still "triggered" in the present, then the wound hasn't healed.

It becomes difficult when dealing with chronic illness as the wound remains open. There are glimpses of hope and normality. Then it emerges again, taking away all shreds of hope at times. Working on the "triggers" to build better coping skills for me has had an immense effect on decreasing "triggers."

CHAPTER 15

PIVOT, DAMN IT! PIVOT!

It seemed like life had progressed and I had not. It had been a very long haul thus far, one that had taken an immense toll on my health, both physically and emotionally. It became blatantly apparent that I had survived but was still in constant survival mode—not living life, just surviving. I had reached a point where I could eat only a handful of whole foods, all being organic. My diet consisted of red potatoes (I could make fries and latkes), white rice, onions, garlic, cauliflower, rolled oats (I could make oatmeal cookies with rice flour), lactose-free and preservative-free butter and cream cheese, eggs, water, and organic coffee. I'm not sure if I can count onions and garlic as whole food items.

I was on self-health management at this point in life. My life involved taking set meds at set times, and I had to up my meds should I want to do or go anywhere, visit anyone, or do anything that involved a change to my activity.

Life became a game of hit and miss. The trial and error of it all costing me weeks at a time in bed, or worse, a ride to the hospital for emergency IV fluids.

As time progressed, I got better at managing it and was keenly aware of the beginnings of a reaction. Extreme reactions left me debilitated for weeks on end. My limited food items became nonexistent, as I had to wait for the degranulation of mast cell and inflammation in my gut to settle. If not, it was like adding gas to a fire.

I had sadly come to the conclusion that this is what the rest of my life was going to look like.

It was depressing, and honestly, I had reached a point of not wanting to live this way. I even uttered the words that I wanted to sign a DNR. I never did, but the words still left my lips as tears left my eyes.

I spent most of my days just trying to stay alive. I became this shell of a person that I used to be. The outgoing and positive person I once was became an extreme introvert and negative.

I was completely and utterly perplexed at how the world, or I should say people in this world, could lack such empathy and compassion, especially for what they could not see. Living with any illness is an incredibly difficult task. I can only speak for myself on living with an invisible illness. At times, it felt like I was floating in the middle of the ocean.

BOBBING UP AND DOWN.

TRYING TO CATCH MY BREATH.

TRYING TO STAY ALIVE.

DROWNING INVISIBLY, RIGHT IN FRONT OF EVERYONE'S EYES!

I can't tell you how many times my husband heard me say, "I just don't understand why they don't get it. Why does it feel to me that those closest to me don't grasp both the severity and scope of my illness? Why do they say the things they say? Why do they lack such empathy?"

Just so we are clear, mast cell patients generally can't eat mainstream foods. We can't, for the most part, consume much of anything, especially most foods that contain histamine, soy, gluten, higher protein content, preservatives, additives, hormones, coloring, and on and on. It's just much easier to say what we can tolerate and eat.

We are hypersensitive to all our surroundings. We can't drink alcohol. We are hypersensitive to smells, be it perfume, candles, smoke, flowers, chemicals. Basically, you name it. So, to someone with mast cell hearing about that awesome dinner you just ate, it's emotionally painful.

We lack the ability to join in. Most individuals who are chronically ill are forced to view life through the eyes of others. To some extent, we cannot join in for a variety of reasons. There's a daily struggle as we receive constant reminders of the life we used to live. Of the person we used to be.

We not only struggle with this emotionally, but there's also an added twist of feeling isolated. Almost all of society socializes with food and alcohol. It matters not what the day has brought. If it's a good day, let's celebrate it with food and drink. Let's reward ourselves; why the hell not? If it's a bad day, let's have a pity party with food and booze. Let's drown our troubles away. If you think about it, every holiday in life pretty much involves food. Food and booze, to a degree, have turned into the drug of choice for many. It is taught from a very young age: Eat your broccoli, and I will reward you with a cupcake for dessert.

Society has lost the art of actually connecting with one another. Some individuals are more interested in what there is to drink and what foods are going to be served. Who is attending is often a secondary thought.

Society has lost the true function of food. It is to fuel our bodies, not to fuel or numb our emotions. I found this to be one of my largest challenges with this disease. Food was my drug of choice, so to speak. I used food, like a lot of people do, to mask emotions, and I had specific foods when I needed to cope with life's challenges. I also had an enabler, my loving husband. If I had a bad day, he knew that Rollo ice cream would pretty much fix it all. When I needed to take the edge off social anxiety or to de-stress, it was with red wine.

I went through what most people go through when they have a sugar and carb addiction—a whopping, nasty withdrawal.

Sugar and heavy carb withdrawal was absolutely horrible on top of being chronically ill.

Headaches, muscle aches, nausea, bloating, irritability. My emotions were on high alert, and I felt completely alone. When I noticed the feelings of being in a down mood deepen, I did what I have done before in life when I felt I was not coping as well as I could be. I sought out help.

I contacted a therapist and booked an appointment. To my surprise and relief, she was helpful. That comment is not a knock at the field of mental health practitioners. It is just an intro to a point I want to make that if you have tried counseling before and didn't find it helpful, possibly give it a go again. I'd had various therapists and counsel in my late teens and then again in my late thirties, but I didn't find it worked for me. I gave it a go again once I researched methods various therapists use. I believe the right match and method was the difference for me.

The right match, from my perspective, needs to be several things:

SOMEONE WHO IS EASY FOR YOU TO TALK TO.

SOMEONE WHO IS QUALIFIED FOR YOUR NEEDS.

SOMEONE WHO OFFERS A VARIETY OF METHODS TO ASSIST YOU; SOMEONE WHO OFFERS DIRECTION FOR SUCCESSFUL COPING SKILLS AND IS WILLING TO EXPERIMENT TO SEE WHICH VARIOUS METHODS WORK THE BEST FOR YOU.

It is a personal experience. Your mindset, triggers, difficulties, and methods for which to cope are as individual as you are. ONE SIZE DOES NOT FIT ALL when it comes to mental health.

If I can say anything else on the subject of mental health, it is this: Mental health assistance in all forms should be easy to obtain, flexible in choice, and affordable to all. It should be part of a paid perk of being human. Now more than ever, proper mental health assistance could benefit mankind. At the least it should be at the top of the list when someone becomes chronically or terminally ill. It should be available for their families and caregivers.

Simply as a form of preventive and self-care, mental health assistance should be a priority in this world, and one that is made easily accessible to all. I would like to think humanity has grown and the stigma has decreased substantially. Perhaps the roadblocks to accessibility and costs should also decrease substantially. I can't think of a better time for humanity's shift in mental health care.

Here and now is the time!

Self-care doesn't fix a flawed you, but it encourages you to embrace the fact that you are already enough. It encourages you to love yourself for who you are—to better yourself with positive coping skills and internal positive narrative.

I'm chronically ill, but I'm also enough just the way I am. Within my own practice and further education, I was capable of nurturing healthier coping skills, which formulated a deeper growth in several areas of my life by developing healthier boundaries.

Being authentic should be a natural state. When an uneasiness creeps in, it signals that you are going against your grain.

I am a confident introvert. I am not an extrovert, which I honestly constantly fought to be throughout my life. Part of that persona was based in my confidence in myself and abilities, so I appeared to be an extrovert to others. In reality, I have always had a manageable amount of social anxiety. I am not a comfortable extrovert—it's against my grain and not authentic.

I don't mind being alone with myself. In fact, I rather enjoy it to a degree. It allows me to write, paint, practice yoga, meditate, and lose myself in a richly rewarding book. It's what allowed my newfound passion of DNA and genealogy to flourish. That particular passion didn't emerge until I became chronically ill, when I taught myself all about this theory of math, ratios, and data and how it related to DNA, lineage, and history. DNA is numbers—and numbers make sense to me. They are straightforward and predictable. I created my own system of bio-tracing and implemented it with success, which gave me a purpose. It kept my mind active while being housebound and bedridden. It also introduced me to others who had the passion or had the need for assistance. Bio-tracing someone's DNA allows me to let someone know who their biological family is and how they are connected. I have done approximately forty-plus cases so far for individuals looking to find their family roots. It fuels me with purpose and is immensely rewarding. The trust others bestow to me with their DNA, with their journey, and with their life's quest is such an honor. It brings me great joy to be of service, and it fits with me being a confident, natural introvert.

But for those who are true extroverts with a chronic illness, the isolation could be a much deeper transition and could cause a darker level of despair.

While attending counseling, my therapist keenly congratulated me in formulating new coping skills without using the crutch of food to mask emotions. I had never really looked at it that way. Yes, it was true that when faced with a really bad day, I wanted nothing more than to eat a plate of pasta. But that and any amount of countless other foods would cause me to be deathly ill, so I had to relearn how to feel that emotion and work through it.

It was the "feeling" part that I had difficulty with. I did not like to actually feel sad or angry or experience fear, but I can't say that anyone really does.

Food used to be my comfort, and when food was forcefully removed from my life, so were my coping skills. It's been a work in progress with many ups and downs and many successes and meltdowns along the way.

To my surprise and shock, some friends and family added more to the struggle of this area of life. They would openly say, "Oh, it's so good. Too bad you can't eat this." Sadly, some individuals made my overall battle with chronic illness more than difficult and almost unbearable.

Being isolated, I would eagerly pick up the phone to converse with just about anyone. However, I was not saddened when the conversation ended if I had to endure descriptions of what they ate at their favorite restaurant or how much pizza and ice cream cake they had consumed at a get-together or worse, the best wine they had ever tasted.

I would get off the phone and think, *they just don't get it.* They lack an understanding of both my struggle and illness. I would try to repeat specific phrases to Jeff so he could understand why I felt saddened after having conversations with others.

If I knew an individual had severe mobility issues, with say MS, I would never talk to them about an awesome workout I had and how freeing and wonderful it was to be in such great physical shape. And I'd never remark that it was too bad that they couldn't join in. There is so much in this world to talk about, and if people were actually tuned in with others, they would gauge their conversations accordingly. Again, some people lack empathy for what they cannot see.

NOTE TO SELF

Chronic illness happened to me, but everyone else's life carried on with very little change. You cannot expect others around you to change immediately in habitual daily conversations when they have been conversing with you in this manner for many, many years. Give them the benefit of the doubt, as most of the time, they don't mean to hurt your feelings.

TAKE A MOMENT FOR YOURSELF

Breathe, Pause, Reflect . . .

Have there been points of time in your life when you felt so alone, even when you were surrounded by people?

Was the feeling of aloneness related to feeling:

Unheard?

Hopeless?

Detached as life moved on without you?

Getting in touch with the core of our feelings is difficult at times. Understanding the root emotion of your feelings is even more difficult.

You can feel angry. Anger tends to be an easy emotion to feel. Most people are comfortable with that feeling, but generally, there's an emotion that comes before the anger. You could feel helpless, hopeless, sad, fearful, or anxious. These emotions are not so easy to be comfortable with. These are the root emotions that we generally avoid. Healing is understanding the emotion, developing coping skills, and healing at the root. Once healed, the anger will go away on its own.

Be Your Own Beacon

Taken down by an invisible illness,
And still I chose love

Bedridden, broken, filled with hunger and pain,
And still I chose love

Losing a life I once reigned,
And still I chose love

Crawling until I could stand, then walk,
And still I chose love

Verbally, emotionally, and physically beaten down,
And still I chose love

Broken physically and emotionally again and again
And still I chose love

Life filled with challenges and uncertainty
And still I chose love

I am a beacon of light and hope for myself
Because I chose love

CHAPTER 16

THE OAK TREE IS THE ROCK

I sat alone in my solitude, pondering over the events of the last few days. The time had come when a very strong and very funny man would be taking his last breath. He battled his illness like a champ; he was knocked down so many times in life, but he always looked up. He was a testament to endurance and humor. He lived life well and on his own terms. He had his vices, like most of us, but in his true nature, he announced at sixty, "That's it, I am done with smoking." True to his word, he never picked up a cigarette again. Such willpower!

I had looked at my phone at least thirty times during the day, checking messages. I checked to make sure the landline was functioning. I sat and waited for "the call," which was imminent. I had been here before, the pre-mourning dance where the room swirled as thoughts of past and present came crashing together. Emotions and heart rate were both quick to rise. You did your best to balance and swerve the curveball that you knew was headed your way. It's unusual if you do this dance alone, though it does happen. With our family, we were all in different living environments. We're multigenerational, yet we all danced to the same sad song in our own separate way, our own separate style, as needed.

Being here before didn't make it any easier. There were new twists of the unexpected with each loved one who passed. Our family acted exactly how I expected us to. Some buried their heads in the sand, while others acknowledged the situation, all doing their best to manage. For the most part, we'd been supportive, stable with emotions, and predictable. I say for the most part because the pre-mourning dance floor became slippery when our son's girlfriend of two years was insistent that she be allowed to say her goodbyes at his deathbed. A dilemma arose after my fourth attempt failed at being "nice." I am not really sure how many ways one can say, "Gramps was a proud man, and he wanted everyone to remember him the way he was. He didn't even want anyone to see him sick, never mind taking his last breath. Please do not go."

She poured out her emotions over a past death and reasoning that really didn't apply to the situation. Why? Because she was reliving her pain, talking from the wound. Her feelings were valid. She was trying in desperation to grasp hold of a solution so she wouldn't feel such painful regret again. I see that now. She's a survivor. A go-getter. A strong, junior oak tree.

"It's not about you," I said bluntly and factually. Why? Because some people don't like to be told no and will go to great lengths to turn your "no" to a "maybe" to a "yes." Their persistency can wear you down. In reality, it is an attribute that I admire, but in that moment, I was physically exhausted and emotionally drained. I, for one, wasn't having any part of it. My first priority was ensuring Pops had his wishes respected. The best we can do during the pre-mourning dance is to allow everyone to dance it the way they choose. Allow it to flow naturally with the rhythm of life. Hold close joyous memories from the past and wait patiently for our loved one to depart when it is their time to do so. We have bittersweet thoughts that start out as encouragement for the loved one to stay a little longer and end with encouragement for them to let go. The logical oak tree in me knew his vitals and had already put the next steps necessary in my mind's place.

Like most days, I was wearing multiple hats. After a long and emotional day, my hats were slipping at 1:30 a.m. I was trying hard to be the loving, respectful daughter-in-law and the loving, protective mother. I personally do not judge one way or the other as to the necessity of family being at the deathbed, as long as the individual passing did not have an issue with it. The one passing has the right to their request being fulfilled and their feelings validated. The right to dignity. The right to peace of mind that their loved ones will have positive, loving, and happier memories of them.

THE FAMILY OAK TREE

Every family has an "oak tree." You either are one or know one. We are not hard to miss. We are the family member who forms the "glue" that meshes and sometimes shakes up the tree. We are the ones who have invisible shoulders so wide that you would be shocked if they became visible. We are the go-to person. The one who makes things happen, fixes things, and gives logical direction. We are organized! We are direct and sometimes brutally honest; we don't sugarcoat much, as it's not in our nature. True oak trees despise gossip of all forms and people who put down others to falsely elevate themselves. We can easily spot the posers who try to manipulate, and we silently take note. We find it hard to trust, and we rely heavily on facts. I am that person in my family and extended family. I didn't ask to be, it is a force of nature. A mystical gene that emerges on its own as life molds and twists it into shape. It allows you to stretch out your arms to support family and friends somewhat like an enormous oak tree. It doesn't matter how drained the oak tree is, when we are called to family and friend duty, we are there to do what we do best—provide logic and support in healthy ways.

It can be tough being the strong oak. We are judged in many arenas of life, sometimes harshly by the ones we want the most respect and love from: our family. I have been told many a time I am too honest, too blunt. I've had family members say, "I love you because your mine, but I don't like your brutal honesty and other aspects of your personality."

I have been asked many times to sugarcoat something and tell a white lie. I've been called "opinionated" and worse, for that matter. I will not apologize for who I am and that facet of my personality. I, however, have failed in allowing myself to feel disappointed and shamed for who I am. My opinion is rarely given without permission to do so, a trait I had to work at. My honesty, brutal or not, is an attribute. It is no different from the depth of my loyalty, strength, logic, and love. Honesty is highly valued when you agree with someone, but tragically wasted and feared on those who don't really want to hear it. Honesty is someone's opinion. That honesty can be factual, right, wrong, and indifferent. Honesty is not to be confused with arrogance. I, for one, have made mistakes throughout my life, and I have zero issue in saying, "I was wrong, and I apologize."

Honesty can be a fickle friend. Being honest is sometimes the catalyst to being vilified. My thoughts are cast back to a moment in time. Caught between a rock and a hard place, I watched in silence as a close individual's life spiraled out of control with children in tow. I watched in silence as the behind-the-scenes maneuvers and manipulation were attempted by others. I was encouraged by another to take action. My act of an upfront (not behind their back) maneuver, honesty, and tough love was greeted as an act of betrayal. Those eyes did not see the closing troops, nets cast behind their back. Those ears did not want to hear the offer to take care of children, bear the cost of therapy and services, or pay for childcare and education so they could better provide for themselves and their children. Those eyes did not see my pain or the unconditional love at any cost. My upfront honesty was the beginning to the end and cost me the relationship. I was immediately thrown under the bus by the same that encouraged me to take action, then others decided to back the bus over me several times to ensure the point was made. Lessons learned: Some individuals will always show the pattern of getting others to do their dirty work. If it goes well, they are the hero, if not, you are the villain. Having broken bird syndrome when I want to help others, but in the end it detrimentally impacts me needs to stop. Being empathetic with boundaries is healthy. I cannot save the world, and not everyone wants to be saved. Not my monkey, not my circus.

I checked my phone once again and reflected on my attempts to be the family's pillar of strength, their oak tree. My tears began to well and my breathing became shaky as I tried to control emotions that didn't want to be controlled. I was my father-in-law's only girl. I had been since I was fifteen years of age. Now, as a seasoned fifty-two-year-old, I had seen the good, the bad, and the "you have got to be kidding me" stages of his life. He was a dedicated husband, father, and grandfather. All the boys were the apple of his eye, the peanut butter to his jelly. And he loved his wife with all his heart. I was certain his last words would be: "I love you."

We should all be that blessed in life, that loved. It should be said that he never once judged me or told me to sugarcoat a thing. In fact, he would say things that were the total opposite: "Someone needs to run the ship or it will run aground" and "You are a mover and shaker—never apologize for that" and "You unconditionally love my son; he feels loved and happy. I need not want for more."

He didn't just love me because he felt he had to, he respected the core of who I am. He knew if he needed something done, I was his go-to.

I awoke after a restless sleep, feeling tired, tearful, and drained. I checked my phone: no messages. I settled myself down to take in my first cup of coffee, anticipating it might be another long day, when the landline rang. It was barely 9 a.m. My heart pounded in my chest like racing rabbits. It was my mother-in-law. She was calm and composed. "Dick has passed. It happened at 5:35 this morning."

Pops, the man with a wonderful smile, striking blue eyes, and outstanding sense of humor was gone. The date, June 6, 2015, was now tattooed on my heart, along with the dates of others lost. I was the first—and only—family member she called. The sturdy oak tree. She requested that I not notify anyone until the end of the weekend. "Pops wouldn't want his death to ruin everyone's weekend," she said.

I was now put in a position I didn't want to be in. My loyalty card would be played directly against my honesty card. How could I not be honest when faced with family members for the remainder of the weekend? I had two full days of being asked to lie. This totally went against my grain. It was not in my nature. Then it hit: this was not about me. It was about what Pops would have wanted. I was honored that Pops taught me long ago how to present a "poker face," so I would do for him what was necessary out of love, respect, and compassion. I would do it for him, our oak tree, one last time.

NOTE TO SELF

Part of being the oak tree is recognizing the difference and depth of boundaries we need in place for our own mental and physical health. In reality, when Pop passed, I wasn't asked to lie, more so delay telling the truth, the inevitable. The outcome of this moment in time would never change, yet the delay in update would cause no harm and could be timed so no one was traveling with heavy shoulders.

Alignment with values and integrity are honorable. Being flexible, while keeping within alignment, has the ability to deepen oneself in compassion and empathy. Knowing how to balance honesty with compassion and empathy is an art. Timing can be one of the strongest assets in communication—use it wisely.

TAKE A MOMENT FOR YOURSELF

Breathe, Pause, Reflect . . .

Have you ever had a "gut feeling" that went against your grain?

If there was zero detrimental outcome, and you were asked to do it again, would you?

If you said yes and still feel comfortable, then you remain in alignment.

If you said no, then misalignment happened with your choice.

What could you have done differently to keep within your alignment?

A "gut feeling" is real. It is our own beacon to recognizing what feels right for us. It is what guides us in our direction. It is a strength; it is an attribute. Knowing that it is a guide also requires flexibility to change direction and timing, and to gain knowledge. Most of all, it helps you to be your authentic self.

For some, alignment is a word rarely used to describe how we are feeling, thinking, and being, yet it is the best way to describe if we are feeling balanced overall in our life's journey.

Can you think back to another situation that represented a misalignment with whom you are as an individual?

Journaling or self-authoring allows us to dig deep into knowing oneself. Sometimes it gives us answers, solutions, and strategies to better handle our journey forward while keeping within our alignment.

CHAPTER 17

NEXT STEPS

On June 6, 2015, my father-in-law passed away from his hard-fought battle with cancer. It was a loss felt deeply by the entire family. It was a loss that devastated Jeff. His father, Dick, was one of his closest friends. They talked every day, and Jeff cherished the time they spent together.

My father-in-law's death would change not only our family circle but also my husband's state of mind. It was the beginning of a marked change in him. This happy-go-lucky person melted into one of sadness and melancholy. He was filled with anxiety over work, his long hours, and his work truck, and driving for work in the winter literally became impossible. That time also increased his worry about losing me.

He began with lots of weighty questions:

DO I REALLY NEED TO WORK AT THIS POINT?

DO I HAVE ENOUGH MONEY TO RETIRE?

DO I HAVE TO WORK THE WINTERS?

DO WE REALLY NEED THIS BIG OF A HOUSE?

SHOULD I REALLY BE WORKING WHEN YOU ARE SO SICK?

ISN'T MY PLACE HERE WITH YOU, WHILE YOU ARE SICK?

WHAT IF YOU NEED ME WHILE I AM AT WORK?

WHAT IF SOMETHING HORRIBLE HAPPENS TO YOU AND I'M NOT HERE?

WHEN THEY FIND A CURE FOR YOU, DO YOU THINK WE SHOULD TRAVEL?

In truth, I was barely holding onto life by the skin of my teeth. Barely keeping my own shit together. I had always been the strong one in our relationship, the high achiever, the breadwinner. The one that steered the ship. I realized in that moment that even though illness had crept into our marriage, the players were still the same. While I was off trying to stay alive, no one was steering the ship. I needed to figure out life's other obstacles, and I also needed to take back some of my own power. I needed to make decisions I didn't want to make. If there is one thing in life that

I've learned about myself, it's that I'm a woman who hates being backed into a corner. I will avoid the corner at all costs. However, when you are chronically ill, the corner becomes a reality. So, you do your best to not get backed into all the other corners in the room, if you can.

Throughout our marriage, Jeff has always expected me to have life's answers to everything. But this time, I had nothing, nada, zippo, zilch. There's nothing like living life flying by the seat of your pants. Another thing about me, which I am guessing you would have figured out by the previous chapters, is that I like predictability. Hence, that is why my mindset throughout life was linear. Flying by the seat of your pants was like a crash-and-burn predictability for me. I am not a gambling person. For me, living on the edge, being wild and crazy, was a trip to the grocery store with no list in hand.

So, I stalled, and I changed the subject.

"Hey, babe, did I tell you about this remarkable dream? I was in a hospital bed with all our family standing around, and we were all eating pizza to celebrate. I was eating the pizza. What a dream!"

Yes, I even celebrated with food and booze in my dreams. It was the joy of togetherness, of sharing, of bonding. This dream was so real that my mouth watered. Damn, I miss pizza! Not everyone will get this comment, but those who do will know what I mean.

When I awoke from that dream, I could not for the life of me get the damn thing out of my head. When I told my husband about it, we giggled a bit, then we fell sadly silent. The entire feeling of it was so strong. Perhaps it was an inkling of what could be.

By the end of the day, I had received an email detailing the announcement of a new drug treatment for mast cell activation disorder. Bam! Just like that, the hope of the dream came to the realization of a possibility. I wept with joy.

It didn't matter how many times I tried to tell myself not to get too excited, I squealed with happiness at the possibility of having my life back.

It was a turning point, or so I thought. I had to weigh the pros and cons of the medication and the disease and the depth of my disability. I soon realized that the pros and cons became irrelevant, as I no longer wanted to live this life as it was. I thought I was rational in my thought process. I was keenly aware that the pain, mobility issues, and gastroparesis would not go away—they hadn't thus far at least. Neither would other debilitating symptoms. That being said, I would possibly gain the ability to eat and nourish my body and join in meals with family and friends once more, which would nourish my soul.

Concerned family and friends wanted to point out the horrible potential side effects. I kindly thanked them and gave them smiles, pointing out that it could stop my allergic response to foods while also pointing out that the serious side effect of anaphylaxis was death. Well, if no one else was going to be excited about this latest development, I knew who would: Rhonda. I could not wait to forward her the info and chat about the possibilities.

Rhonda and I connected on a Facebook group. Some groups can be a great source of information, while others can be a connection of shared woes and hopes and provide a level of empathy and understanding that others just don't comprehend. Rhonda also has the same double whammy as I do—mast cell and hyper-POTS. In truth, she just isn't one of my closest chronically ill friends, she's one of my closest friends, period. Rhonda always gets it because she's got it! You know what I mean?!

I forwarded her the research and drug name and followed it up with: "I am going to take one for the team. I'm going to be the guinea pig. I am ready! Why, you ask, my dear friend? Mainly because I have lost my patience with it all!"

Patience is not my strongest suit. I've always felt that if I didn't keep pushing for a treatment, a protocol, and management, and keep reading the latest research, then a better quality of life would not be obtained. The gaslighting from others had the opposite effect on me, to a degree. It made me realize once my disease was validated that if I didn't keep pursuing living a fully healthy life and pushing the boundaries in all areas, no one would do it for me. If I wanted to have a life that was more about living than just staying alive, I had to save my own self!

At one point in our close, laughable, cry-your-eyes-out, let's-figure-this-shit-out relationship, we played the game of . . . "You try it first and let me know how it goes."

This time, I put the ball into play first and relatively fast. I promptly gathered all the medical articles I could. I saved them in files and forwarded them to my family physician with a request for an appointment to discuss this potential treatment. I had a three-week wait. Ugh. In reality, that was nothing. Most specialist's appointments were six to eight months out, some even two years out.

The day finally arrived, and I prepared myself for a potential disappointment. But I felt surprisingly hopeful and positive after the doctor's meeting. We were both on the same page. She would start the hunt for a doctor who could administer and manage the treatment plan if they felt I was a good candidate for the medication. Or should I say, if the medication was right for me. I rushed home to contact those I needed to tell: Rhonda and Jeff. Rhonda really got me and understood exactly what I was going through, and I mean all of it. And Jeff always gave me such unconditional love and support. At that point in my world, others who should have or could have been in the loop were not.

My adult children have always been great support, but I kept a lot of my serious issues, including the possibility that it might be cancer, hidden from them. I was always being their mom, protecting them from worry. I tried to smile when it was painful. Smile when I was emotionally beaten down. Smile and say, "I'm good. I'm fine." I tried as hard as I could to give them a glimpse of the old mom pre-chronic illness that I could muster up. Sometimes, most times, it was extremely draining to keep up the charade. I called it the "fake happy face."

My gut told me this potential new treatment would be a rough ride and that maybe I should call in reinforcements for this part of my journey. But first, I decided to wait until I heard back from my family physician as to the next step. Until then, I would do my best to remain hopeful and positive.

The wait time to get back in to see the immunologist was painful and emotional. I arrived full of hope and determination and left feeling crushed and defeated. He said there was no way in hell he would prescribe the new medical treatment because the risks were just too high.

His words just kept repeating in my head like a loop, over and over. No new medication. No new treatment for me. It was loud and clear. I felt devastated and hopeless.

Over that year, life turned into a blur. There was so much happening in my life that it would have been difficult for a non-chronic individual to keep up. I had no career, and I was forced to sell off my book of business. I was also forced to negotiate this deal with the manager who bullied me at the end of my career. I had expressed deep concerns to HR in an email requesting I deal with other management to formalize the selling of my book of business, but it fell on deaf ears.

He bullied me through the entire process. It was a horribly defeating time in my life, a time in which I had to endure his abuse of power and control. I lost my career and the perks that went along with it. After the perks ran out, I was quickly and abruptly fired from my twenty-two-plus years of loyal service in the banking industry. It did not matter that I had a pristine HR record. I was just a number to them. The firing was another huge blow. The letter and paperwork that followed indicated I was fired out of "frustration." They were frustrated that I could not return to work in my capacity or fill another capacity. I was chronically ill, and they were the ones claiming frustration.

WTF?!

You're probably asking, "Can they do that legally?" The answer is yes, they can, and in most instances, they probably will. They have a business to run. I was merely a worker bee who disrupted the hive. Survival of the fittest. I was just a number. You think that I would have figured that out right from the beginning when they gave me my employee number.

I was backed into another corner yet again. Money was tight, and Jeff wanted to move. He had stopped working winters at that point. I rationalized that we really didn't need a house as big as our four-bedroom split-level. We rarely used the family room. Dinner in the dining room had become nonexistent since I fell ill. Two of the four bedrooms were converted—one into a den, the other into the dogs' bedroom and an overflow closet. Yes, you read that correctly. The dogs (there were three at that point) all had sleeping crates in their own bedroom. The third bedroom was a guest room. The basement was used by Jeff when hockey was on, but the pool table was covered in dust and the exercise equipment held nothing but memories and clothing that came out of the dryer damp. Our huge outdoor entertainment area sat vacant most times, and the pool cost us one thousand dollars to open and another thousand to close without getting used once in the previous year. I felt forced in many ways to sell the family home we'd had for more than two decades. It was our forever home. I had lovingly fixed it up just the way we wanted. It held all the memories of our children growing up. All the holiday meals and parties, all the Sunday family dinners and gatherings. It was home. They say, "Home is where your heart is." Well, my heart was there, and at times, it still is. The hub of the Kewell family was no more. It was a done deal.

Packing and purging was tiring and heartbreaking. It brought forward a life I had cultivated that no longer existed. It was the start of the next pivot, although at the time, I didn't realize it. It was a forced pivot in all aspects, yet it turned into a conscious one of growth. I had to make decisions about moving. I had to get rid of excess stuff. I had to purge.

The word "purging" as a noun means "purification of cleansing."

KEEP.

SAVE.

LET GO.

I am not going to lie or sugarcoat this. It was emotionally painful, not just for me but also for Jeff. In a lot of areas of the home, it was actually harder for Jeff.

It was a shitty buzz. And it was brutal at times.

I had left some things until the last possible moment. Hidden in the basement laundry room were several boxes. Honestly, I had never even touched them when they entered our home while I was critically ill. They were the three boxes a stranger had dropped off—unannounced—from a delivery service. His only words had been, "Sign here."

I had asked Jeff to move them to the back of the laundry room, and they became out of sight, out of mind. Those three boxes held what felt like was my entire career. They held my education diplomas and prized certificates, so nicely framed. They held wonderful memories; they held part of my identity. It took me a full day to complete the purge. The first box wasn't too bad because it contained desk items that held no memories other than their use: pens, paper, sticky notes. Credenza items were filtered among the remnants and held similar value. But when I opened the second box, it was a whole new ballgame of emotions. Cherished photos of my boys, of work trips, of fundraising golf tournaments. My life in pictures—a life I no longer lived.

I paused the purging only to grab tissues, catch my breath, and find my courage to go on.

I sat motionless at the top of the stairs, looking at the boxes.

The neatly folded hard edges just waiting to give me a paper cut to the bone. It was like salt on my wounds. I summoned up the courage and yelled at the top of my lungs, "Rip the Band-Aid off, damn it. Just rip that sucker right off!"

My warrior cry rang out and echoed off the bare basement walls.

I purged and cried and purged some more. I formed a rhythm with my motions, robotic and with intent.

KEEP.

SAVE.

LET GO.

KEEP.

SAVE.

LET GO.

DONE AND DONE!

NOTE TO SELF

Expand my passions for my love of education. Update my coaching certification. Further my certifications in the areas of trauma, chronic illness, and well-being. It's time to regenerate my mind and reinvest in myself. Healing the body as a whole heals the human spirit.

Expand on my creative areas that bring me peaceful moments, such as my writing, photography, painting, yoga, meditation, and breath work.

MUSKOKA LIFE

I realized that Muskoka is the right place to start the new part of my journey. The gorgeous remote area north of Toronto is dotted with lakes and peppered with trees and breath-taking scenery. There, at our cottage, I will be able to pause and breathe.

It took months for Jeff and me to complete the purge of twenty-two years' worth of life. The move to our cottage required a lot of work and emotional strength for which I put on a fake happy face. It required a renovation to make it a healthy place, as there were some water issues to be resolved.

Just like Superman's downfall was kryptonite, mine was any form of mildew or mold. It was a huge expense to remediate, but it needed to be done. It also added a huge amount of stress personally, as well as to our marriage. Jeff was now out of work full time, and our worries seemed endless. We had to hire lawyers to recover moneys owed, but almost half went to legal fees. Between that, the renovations, and my health issues, it was a stressful time.

The transition to the cottage was chaotic. We had placed money down on a condo near our old home as a safety net in case things didn't go as planned. It was a lot when coupled with my health issues that still had no real answers, no cures, and no management in place at all, unless you call doing your own research online a form of health management. For all those reading this who are thinking that it couldn't be that bad, I assure you, I am not the only one who feels this way. There are others who live with the struggle of not only getting a proper diagnosis in a reasonable amount of time but of also not getting assistance in managing and treating the chronic illness so they can live a better quality of life. I am not alone. There are, unfortunately, way too many warriors with the same struggles.

I tried to do my best to socialize when we moved. I also kept busy with my hobbies and passions. To this day, they still keep me going.

By late fall 2016, my health had reached an all-time low. I weighed in below 100 pounds again! My weight had varied over the course of my illness. It was up. It was down. I hoped there wouldn't be any talk again of tube feeding.

My blood work came back with forty-six labs abnormal. Crap! Suddenly it was like the medical support I did have in place went into panic mode. I had been chronically ill since 2012, so why the big panic now? I guess forty-six abnormal labs warranted a degree of urgency.

It was if the doctors all woke up and said, "Holy shit, there is something seriously wrong here."

They rushed to get me into a hematologist, but it wasn't a direct route there. The day before my appointment, I collapsed in Toronto on my way to the hospital lab to get more blood work done and wound up in the emergency department.

That night spent in the ER was an eye opener. Have you ever

been to a busy emerg during a full moon? It's really something else. I shit you not.

Some patients were in their own open cubicle; others, like me, were all pushed together in the larger open area of the room. The cubicle over my right shoulder had two police officers sitting patiently waiting, for what I did not know. I had been there for several hours when I told Jeff to go back to our son's condo, as it was going to be a long night, and rather than just sit in the waiting room, he'd be more comfortable at Jason's. After all, it was right across the street. He was reluctant but eventually agreed.

An hour later, all hell broke loose in the ER. A young man began running wildly around the room, wearing nothing but a hospital gown open in the back and showing his bare ass. He was screaming at the top of his lungs, "Catch me if you can! Catch me if you can!"

At first, I found it slightly comical. He seemed somewhat childlike and nonthreatening as he ran like the wind, laughing and grabbing anything and everything he could. Then his facial expression turned dark, and he lost his innocent grin as he began knocking over trays, pans, and grabbing people's belongings. He violently threw anything in his path as he ran between the gurneys.

"You'll never catch me, bitchhhhhh!" His words hissed as he glared down the nurse from four feet away.

He spun around, knocking metal food trollies to the polished terrazzo flooring. Green Jell-O, oatmeal, and apple juice flew in multiple directions. It was the distraction he wanted. He hurdled over the few seats in the room, outmaneuvering the staff with ease. He was quickly moving in my direction with two nurses and security following closely. Would the security guards get to him before he got to me? That was my burning question.

I lay there motionless, trying to make myself invisible as I pulled the cotton sheet up to my chin, trying not to draw attention to myself. I looked up at my oxygen and IV hanger. I was trapped. Shit, shit, shit—I couldn't get out of bed, never mind try to run. Our eyes made contact, and I knew in that moment that it wasn't going to end well.

He was steps away from the end of my bed when his eyes shifted to my bright red winter jacket. His hands reached to grab it when he abruptly came to a crashing halt as a male nurse stepped in between the running man and my bed. The patient was quickly subdued and slightly sedated, then harnessed to a bed to my right for the protection of all. He was resting peacefully within minutes.

Me, not so much. My heart was pounding at over 130 beats per minute according to the monitor.

Man, it was a long night. I was afraid to shut my eyes, let alone sleep.

More blood tests were ordered. Scans needed to be done. The emerg doctor indicated that I needed to be watched overnight, as my tests showed potential blood clots in my lungs, macrocytic anemia, which the doctor felt the hematologist would be better suited to discuss in the morning at my scheduled appointment.

It was now two in the morning. I wasn't sure if I should call Jeff because he was probably sleeping. Just then, I received a text from him. It was if he had been thinking of me at the same time.

> Hey, babe, how's it going? How are you doing? Any news? Love you 😍

> Hi, babe, hanging in there. Why are you not sleeping? Love you too 😍

> Can't sleep. I should have just stayed there with you.

> I have to stay overnight. Come in the morning. Get yourself coffee and a bagel. Can you bring me my organic coffee in a to-go mug and my oatmeal cookie?

> Your wish is my command, my babe. I will be there bright and early. Love you 😍

> Thanks! Love you too 😍

There was no point telling him about the blood clots or the scary running man.

I settled in, thinking I just had to get through this night. After all, what else could happen? I shouldn't have even thought that thought. It was if I asked the universe to give me an up-close look at "shit's getting real now."

I could hear screaming coming from the double emergency room doors. I sat up in my hospital gurney and looked in the direction of the screams. Others in the ward area looked as well. I am sure they felt as I did: WTF is happening now?! I felt like I was on a movie set of the making of a horror movie. Seriously, what the hell was going on now?

The emergency room doors burst open as a gurney was pushed in with full force. Doctors, nurses, EMS rushed in. I could not keep track of the number of moving parts and people. A nurse sat on top of a patient, giving compressions and counting loudly. Another held a mask that pumped air into the patient. They quickly wheeled the gurney over to my left. I watched as the nurse jumped off the patient and yelled, "Clear!"

It was like a train wreck. I didn't want to watch, but I couldn't help myself from looking. Unable to turn my head away, I watched in horror as a doctor literally stabbed a needle into the man's chest with full force. They all rushed around this patient, hooking up wires and machines. I watched the doctor rub the paddles together: "Clear!"

All attending yelled back: "All clear!"

Boom went the paddles. The patient's body partially lifted off the gurney.

My own body jerked at the shock of it all. I felt like I was holding my breath waiting to hear that heart monitor blip into rhythm. Time ticked by.

"Clear!"

"All clear!"

This time, I tightly closed my eyes as my body jerked again to the sound of the defibrillator. Time ticked on. Then the blip, blip, blip of the heart monitor.

Holy shit, they did it! The team pulled off a miracle right before my eyes. Oh, God, the stress they must have been feeling. The rush of adrenaline must have been pumping through their veins. They are heroes without capes. The man and his family would be overjoyed that his life was saved.

They partially closed his curtain at that point. The emergency ward finally started to settle down a bit by 3:30.

A nurse came over to check on me. He took my vitals and made small talk about the craziness that comes out with the full moon. He smiled and raised his nose into the air while sniffing. He leaned toward the person behind me and sniffed again. Quietly, the nurse pushed my gurney forward about three feet away from the man behind me.

"Girlfriend, no one should be subjected to that dirty body odor. I gotcha," he said as he waved his hands in the air, turning to give me a wink.

"You're up," he said to the running man as he released the breaks on his bed and rolled the gurney out for the orderly to safely take him to a designated secured floor. The running man didn't leave quietly.

He pointed at me as he passed by, announcing loudly, "Bitch, that red coat is mine. Whatcha doin' with my coat? Bitch, that red coat is mine before the night is over."

I was still awake at 5 a.m. and somewhat terrified to shut my eyes. In the latest commotion with the running man, I must have missed the arrival of a family member or friend of the man whose life was saved. I glanced over, looking, but trying not to look. I was beyond shocked. The man was sitting up in bed and arguing with the person in his cubicle. I watched him slide out of the bed naked as he ripped out his IV.

I was gob smacked. The man had literally been dead on arrival hours ago. Seriously, what the hell?!

He put on his jeans and his shirt. His visitor stepped in front of him, trying to calmly coach the resuscitated man back into bed.

"You OD'd, man. You gotta stay here. Let them make arrangements for rehab. Let them help you." At first, the visitor pleaded and begged. He then finally demanded, "Get your fucking ass back into that bed!"

The resuscitated man pushed hard on his visitor's chest. "I need a hit, right now. Get the fuck outa my way!"

He left the emergency room almost as quickly as he came in. I watched in disbelief as he pretty much skipped through the double doors.

I was speechless. It was all so surreal; it felt like a movie. I really wanted it to be a bad dream, more for his sake than mine. I desperately wanted someone to yell "Cut!" and wake me.

It was by far one of the wildest nights of my life.

When Jeff arrived that morning, he smiled as he handed me my coffee and cookie. Jokingly, he said, "So, did I miss any excitement last night not being here?"

I just shook my head and rolled my eyes. I didn't even know where to start.

"You are not going to believe it. Honestly, if I didn't see it all with my own eyes, I wouldn't have believed what went on." I sounded exhausted yet oddly wired from my experience that night.

The story would have to wait, as I was being wheeled up to the hematology department with all my results to add to my existing referral.

The panel of blood was shocking to the specialist. She didn't even know how I was functioning. My levels were so low, she didn't know how I could formulate a complete sentence. The blood results indicated that they needed to investigate and rule out more things, very serious things (like the big C). They were now concerned it was cancer.

A bone marrow biopsy, GI scope, and colonoscopy were ordered, along with steroids and a B12 injection, which they scheduled to be done all at the same time in January 2017. The immediate best case would be if the B12 was successful, we could then avoid a blood transfusion. Results would take six to eight weeks.

"Meh," I said to Jeff. "Six to eight weeks is easy-peasy."

I worked with my therapist through the entire process, although it didn't seem to lessen my anxiety over the fear about cancer.

To make matters worse, my beloved Yorkie Abby was diagnosed with cancer during the same six-to-eight week wait. It was too much. I didn't want to talk about it, hear about it, or think about it. I didn't even care how much surgery or treatment cost. I just didn't care. After discussion with our vet, we all decided that if it was operational and the tumor could be cleanly removed, we'd go ahead. If not, we would go in and say our goodbyes. My heart just couldn't take anymore. Jeff and I both felt so beaten down in life at that point in time. It was heartbreaking. Our beautiful, sweet, funny Abigail. She needed to live. I needed her to live now more than ever. The thought of losing Abby was just too much. Losing Abby would always be too much.

Well, I was wrong. I jinxed myself making the statement of "easy-peasy." The wait for my results was horrifically stressful for both Jeff and me. The saving grace was that the results arrived at six weeks, rather than eight.

TAKE A MOMENT FOR YOURSELF

Breathe, Pause, Reflect . . .

Have you ever experienced the loss of a fur baby?

Some individuals describe the depth of grief they feel for a beloved pet to be more heartfelt than the loss of a person they knew. I felt that way and still do, to a degree.

Have you ever given thought as to why the depth of grief of a fur baby has such a huge impact on our journey?

The answer to that is our pets provide us with "unconditional love." It is one of the purest loves there is; they love us without judgment. Unconditional love means never yielding to express all our vulnerabilities, hopes, dreams, and pain.

CHAPTER 18

PIVOTING WITH GRACE

I was filled with gratitude that everything came back negative. Cancer, as well as some other serious diseases, were ruled out. Also on the bright side, the steroids had worked and the B12 was successful. Blood tests showed a slight improvement of my anemia as well. So, things were heading in the right direction with my health crisis, so to speak.

There was a caveat to this moment in time. I didn't realize that a pivotal moment was in play for several areas of my life. I didn't see it coming. It was yin and yang, both being contrary yet interconnected forces in my world. I would only first feel the yin seeping into and invading my life. There were moments that started out leaving me exasperated, then shifted to pure emotional exhaustion, taking the breath out of me. I felt blindsided and devastated, like I was being kicked while down.

I have always prided myself on being "the rock" for others in their time of need, the one who would step up and help. I'm the one who people call when they need a logical answer or advice. I'm the one they can call at 3 a.m. for a breakup or trip to an emergency room. I am that person. Jokingly, I'm the one if a loved called and said, "So, I have this body . . . ," my reply would be "Let me get my shovel." When you are "the rock," people are used to you being that rock. They are used to you fulfilling that niche in their lives.

Right now, I was not HER! I needed someone else to step up be it, her or him! Take your pick, I don't care, it was just somebody else's turn to be "the rock." It was my turn to have someone be "MY ROCK!" The bone marrow biopsy period of time was by far one of the scariest and worst times in my life. I was deathly ill. I was filled with fear and anxiety, and the horrible images of my sister Nancy's last days and last breaths haunted me in my sleep.

I NEEDED TO BE LOVED.

I NEEDED TO BE HUGGED.

I NEEDED TO BE SUPPORTED IN A LOVING KIND OF WAY.

I needed people close to me to have understanding for what I had already gone through in life so far, especially for everything that I had lost due to chronic illness.

I needed them to show empathy. More so, I needed compassion.

I needed individuals to understand and really grasp the fact that I was suffering and grieving the unthinkable, a loss of life. Yes—A Loss of Life!

I was grieving the loss of myself, of my future, of my life as I knew it.

Would it had been too much to ask for some individuals to give me grace?

During my journey being chronically ill, could I have responded or dealt with life in a different way?

Could I have sugarcoated my life and my words more?

Could I have suppressed my anger, sadness, fear, anxiety, and desperation more than I had?

Could or should I have tried harder to cope better?

I was doing the best I could with what coping skills I had at that time. To some, it wasn't enough.

Sadly, to some, I have never been, nor will I ever be, enough. To others, I am just too much.

I've always been and always will be accountable for my words and actions in life. This time was no different.

Was it too much to ask for the same level of accountability?

I have grown as an individual since then. I am more

knowledgeable, and I better see the flags or warning signals. I understand trauma response and the patterns.

I no longer feel the need to over explain, defend, or reason.

Fight or flight are familiar trauma responses, but freeze (not being able to act) and fawn (oversharing, with the opposite side of fawn being over explaining) are less known. Fawn is one that a lot of people resort to in order to avoid conflict. I often found myself fawning when I felt that others weren't understanding my feelings or my difficulties.

Over explaining as a trauma response is explaining something to an excessive degree. It is responding to someone using words, examples, and facts in an attempt to reinforce your point. It holds a level of desperation to be understood, to be heard, and to be listened to. The response causes your body to fall into a negative anxiety loop. Over explaining is a learned cycle that falsely creates a barrier of intellectual protection. It is an ingrained signal used in response while unconsciously trying to control the signal of anxiety.

Oversharing, the opposite to over explaining, is a trauma response generally involving intensity-addiction bonding (basically drama), low self-esteem, loneliness, and victim mentality. The response causes a false high, leading eventually to a negative anxiety loop. It holds a level of desperation to raise self-esteem while tearing down others, bonding in a negative way, and reinforcing the victim mentality.

My patterned behavior was of over explaining rather than oversharing, but it's not who I am. It is a trauma response, a behavior, and therefore, it can be changed.

To break the cycle, one needs to become aware of the pattern, signal, or flag. One needs to recognize that the toxic response is to a toxic processing, to a toxic root cause. Breaking the cycle takes five steps: gather, reflect, right it, reach, and active reach.

Deconstructing the trauma response to understand why one is over explaining or oversharing, then reconstructing a new automated response takes roughly sixty days of reaffirmation to build a stronger, better, and healthier mind and response center.

I also have an ingrained trauma pattern of "ultra-independence." This behavior is acting as if you have everything under control all the time. It's generally a protective behavior constructed so you don't have to ask for help for fear of being perceived as weak or vulnerable. Again, it's a cycle and generally stems from your own experiences in life.

Having trauma response patterns of over explaining and ultra-independence already ingrained prior to illness did not make my journey any easier. Chronic illness brought my actual trauma responses to light. The light allowed me to gather and reflect. Where there is light and recognition, there can be acknowledgment to right it, reach, and active reach.

Acknowledgment and changed behavior bring the opportunity for growth and the power to make better choices. Better choices also generally involve boundaries.

NOTE TO SELF

Dr. Maya Angelou once said, "When people show you who they are, believe them the first time."

This is a difficult lesson to learn, and one that's even harder to implement in life. Individuals who offer anything else but love, understanding, and kindness in your time of need do not nurture your soul. Their behavior shows more of who they are and where they are in that point in life. Growth is acknowledging it and working to change that negative behavior.

Perhaps you are in therapy to deal with the people in your life who don't or won't go to therapy. Who don't or won't change their negative actions toward you.

Growth is having empathy for an individual and understanding their toxic behavior has an underlying trauma. Growth and respect mean *also having empathy for yourself to understand you no longer need to be subjected to the toxic behavior.*

It is not only okay, but also necessary for healthy relationships to break toxic cycles.

You will not only survive, but you will also thrive. Wear your broken-heart badge with honor and shout to the universe: "I am the cycle breaker!"

TAKE A MOMENT FOR YOURSELF

Breathe, Pause, Reflect . . .

My trauma response became more pronounced as my illness progressed. I wasn't even aware I had any trauma responses prior to illness.

Do you have behaviors and patterns that have increased?

If so, digging in deeply to explore these patterns in some cases can provide growth, understanding, acknowledgment, and emotional healing.

Rage

The fire burns within
It rages and scorches all in its path

The fire burns within
It rages on using hate as fuel

The fire burns within
Uncontrollable anger ignites
Setting oneself on fire, expecting others to die from smoke inhalation

The fire burns within
Sensing once the fuel of hate is gone
Reality will appear, forcing her to acknowledge her deep-seated pain

Toxic

You are full of shit. Get some help. It's your fault; you started it. The wrong is all on you. Keep it real. You hurt everyone and everything around you. You are so emotional. You are so sensitive. You are nothing more than an angry person. You are pathetic. You are a depressed bitch. My opinion is right. You don't listen to me. You are a bitch. Did I tell you you're pathetic? Keep it real and skip the physiological mumbo jumbo bullshit. You have no one else on your side. I am your biggest supporter. You had the best of everything, now you don't, so Get Over It. You can't handle anything. This is your wake-up call, so get your shit together. You misinterpret everything. You take everything personally. You hate being called out on anything. You are so pathetically broken. I am here if you ever decide to mend. I can't have anything to do with you if you won't listen to me. You are a horrible person. Just get over it. You are a real bitch. Your words hurt. No one wants to hear what you have to say. No one is even listening to you, so don't bother to speak. You need to take my opinion, but you don't, so it's all on you. You are crazy, batshit crazy. Everything is all your fault. You think you are so much better and smarter than everyone else.

Expectations

When people fail to meet our expectations in who we need and want them to be . . . it is because we failed ourselves in recognizing they are incapable of being that individual. When someone shows you their true colors, believe it . . .

Don't waste time trying to repaint them.

CHAPTER 19

LIVE BLOOD

I love a great mystery. I thrive on the hunt and solving the unknown. The logical side of my brain loves to connect the dots with data, research, and facts, keeping all emotion out of the equation. I must say, figuring out the puzzle of chronic illness was not up there on my bucket list. It was also much harder to keep emotion out of the equation.

I was still trying to crack the puzzle. We know what I didn't have as far as disease and illness were concerned. The symptoms were vast and involved at times.

At this point in time, Ehlers-Danlos syndrome had been taken off the table. So, a genetic illness was not the underlying disease. This was the direction from the specialist's clinic that saw more individuals with EDS in one day than most mainstream doctors would see in their lifetime. The specialist and I were on the same page. The "why" or "where" my illness came from was more than likely viral or bacterial.

Various specialists with backgrounds based in their specific fields have found no regular signs of autoimmune. They had all said it sounds and looks to be autoimmune, but without antibodies, biomarkers, there was no confirmation.

The endocrinologist was puzzled and felt it was going to show up as thyroid; it did not. What it did show through blood tests was that my thyroid was borderline low. I was also confirmed as hypoglycemic; my blood sugar was a four. My temperature was also low, sitting regularly at 96 degrees F (the baseline standard is 98.2 degrees F).

I had been to several naturopaths and functional medicine doctors. I even went as far as to have a "live blood" analysis. I chose to go that route after research on the topic. It was out of the normal scope of medical tests and was not covered by my medical provider. But it was not overly expensive, so why not?

I went in with an open mind, but I still remained my skeptical self. I wanted to see the facts, so I refused to fill out the questionnaire about my health issues because I wanted them to have zero information about me before the test. I wanted them to give me an unbiased report of their findings.

It was an eye opener, to say the least.

Their findings indicated the possibility of chronic Lyme disease from approximately ten years prior, as well as Epstein Barr. They also found mycoplasma and possibly another co-infection. They concluded that a viral or co-infection was still wreaking havoc on my immune system. As to what the viral actually was, though, was undetermined. They literally could see my immune system struggling with inflammation. I marched out of the appointment, feeling bewildered yet vindicated. Then the reality of the results set in. I felt overwhelmed, but hopeful. I also felt cautious as to with whom I would share this information.

When I use the "they," it is because I went to two different sources to have the live blood taken and analyzed. They were not affiliated in any way. Yet they both came back with the same results.

Why was I cautious to share the information? Well, the testing was not mainstream and therefore not taken seriously by most mainstream medical professionals. I really had to ask myself if the chronic Lyme disease and Epstein Barr could have been fluke answers. Mycoplasma is not a common term just thrown around, and I had mycoplasma pneumonia at the age of sixteen. As well, the possible viral damaging my immune system seemed to line up to my being very ill in 2006.

I decided to send the pictures of the live blood to the hematologist to ask her opinion. She indicated that this was not her forte, and I needed an infectious disease specialist. It ended there.

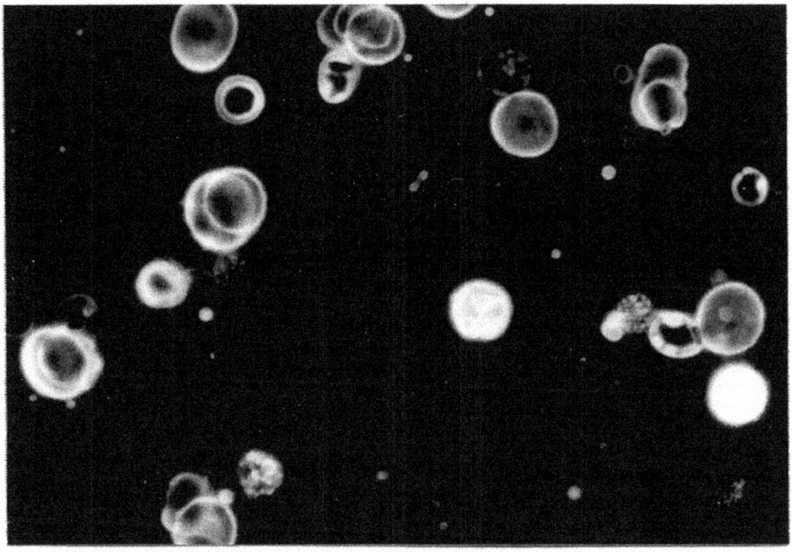

Live Blood File Photos

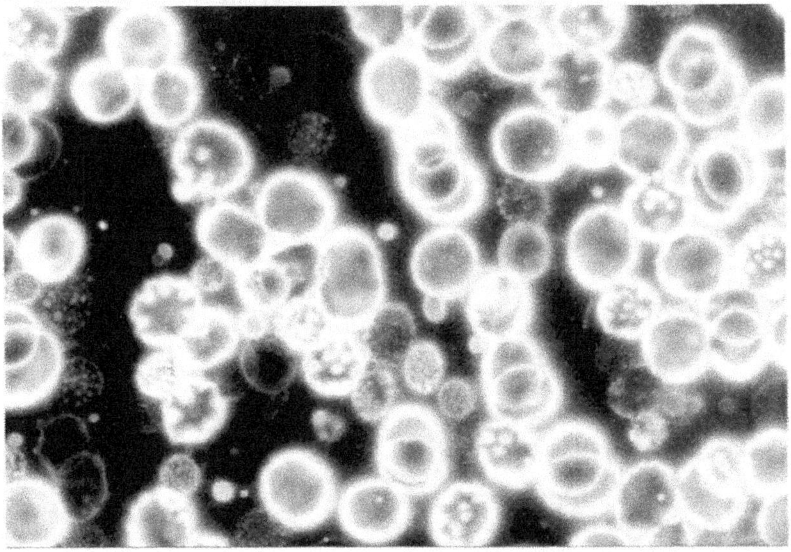

I was to continue with the Cetirizine, Zantac, Benadryl, and 50 mg of prednisone once per month to get the B12 shot in. As I waited for a naturopath appointment to see if the "live blood" would result in a different outcome, my attacks ramped up with spring in full bloom. My body does not like the change of seasons, or weather. When my natural allergies act up, so do my symptoms.

Most of the time I felt like I was left hanging in the wind the moment I left a specialist's office. Like a wet sheet on a blustery day, tangled up on the line. There was still no management of my diagnosed illness as secondary, so I needed to keep looking for the primary.

Feeling frustrated, sick, and not knowing what or who to believe, I went to two other NP and MD offices to have live blood analyses done again. Each time I went, I gave them no information about any previous illness. Just name and age. All three tests came back with the same results: all three showed an attack to my immune system. But trying to get the broad medical community to support these results was something of a mountain-moving experience.

I was left feeling disappointed yet again that there wasn't someone who could shed more light on the underlying cause to this mast cell activation or chronic inflammatory response or idiopathic environmental illness or multiple chemical sensitivity. To me, it was all the same. The key was that there was an underlying cause that made my body go into a hypersensitivity/inflammatory response. I am not a doctor, but I was able to connect the dots and see an overlap of reasonable probability.

My mind raced over notes and the research to find a balance between living a life and simply existing. My sense of humor was still very much alive as I tinkered with ideas way outside the box to weed out the illness. To take it from its hiding spot from within and nudge it to the light of day, so I could then banish it for evermore. I laughed at my creative mind wishing I lived at Hogwarts.

The logical side of my brain would never allow it and would say, "Nope, not happening." But then my adventurous side would counter with: "Why the hell not?!"

My brain and body were tired. I was sick of being sick. I was horrifically tired of explaining and having to justify my "invisible" illness to ANYONE! Their lack of understanding and empathy based on their level of perception didn't help. Some tried; they really did. Others would say they were trying, but they judged and criticized. Some were just downright toxic. It's been bittersweet to let some people and some things go. It comes with the realization that nothing lasts forever. The truth of the matter is that you can't miss a great relationship if it wasn't great to begin with.

There was the heartache and grieving of losing myself and the life I'd envisioned, as well as the pain of losing others before their actual passing. The burning truth is that it's incredibly hurtful and disappointing when others don't meet our expectations of who we need them to be, mainly respectful and kind people. To not cast shame upon us when we're sick and vulnerable. To not be verbally or emotionally abusive. To not constantly judge and criticize and bully.

NOTE TO SELF

If there are issues or cracks in your relationship with others prior to chronic illness, chances are that they'll only be magnified afterward. They will fragment into a million pieces. Set boundaries and protect yourself. Boundaries are not made with the purpose of making another enraged, agitated, or resentful. They are not a grudge. They are to protect the individual setting them and any form of relationship that is left to be saved. Boundaries are a saving grace. Use your grace!

TAKE A MOMENT FOR YOURSELF

Breathe, Pause, Reflect . . .

Setting boundaries is part of self-care. Would your mental and physical health improve if you set boundaries with certain individuals in your life?

If so, do you think you can establish those boundaries?

If not, perhaps seek out assistance to formulate a strategy on how to place boundaries that would have the best outcome for your mental and physical health.

CHAPTER 20

LIFE AND DEATH

In 2018 there were doctors' appointments of a joyful nature for a different person in the family. Jeff and I learned that we were to be grandparents for the first time. This wonderful news gave me a boost to push forward and become more assertive in my quest for answers and treatment.

Then, as if the universe answered my quest, a scientific article came across my path. It was a magical lightbulb moment for me as I read it and reread it. Further research confirmed that my type of hyper-POTS had a high rate of being autoimmune-related. I felt gob smacked and validated at the same time.

I did not waste any time and quickly wrote an email to my three main doctors: my family doctor, my immunologist, and my integrative care doctor. I attached the article and requested feedback and possible treatment steps.

I waited with patience. Well, patience is not my best personality trait, I will be honest. I waited one week, then two weeks without a reply. By week three, I resent my email, indicating that this was my second request for a response. I practiced deep breathing and congratulated myself for being patient as the weeks passed. Week four, week five, week six . . . nothing! Being my own health advocate, I started making calls. The integrative care doctor wanted me to follow up with my immunologist.

I finally booked an appointment with my family doctor to discuss the scientific article and potential treatment. My appointment was a two-and-a-half-hour drive from the lake house. I made the long trek down to get the ball rolling. We agreed that a letter would go off to my immunologist in the hopes that my upcoming appointment would focus on looking for the antibodies to confirm autoimmune and a potential treatment.

Weeks passed, and I tried not to focus on the timeline delay. At that point in my illness and dealing with extensive wait times to see specialists, a few months' wait was nothing. I'd learned the hard way that delays and wait times came as part and parcel of the process. I've had wait times up to two years to get in to see a specialist. I was extremely thankful and full of gratitude for every doctor who truly tried to help me and give treatment. From my personal experience and perspective, the wait times and lack of management was a flaw in the medical system. Sometimes, though, I swear the waiting part was a learning lesson, or should I say the lesson of the sickness was to teach me patience? It was, for me, a part of the reasoning. What did others do? The individuals who aren't as stubborn, strong, assertive, and damn well resilient as I am? We're not all capable of being advocates. I worried that if I didn't push on to get answers, no one would.

I worried for those patients who accept the first or third or fifteenth explanation about their health crisis that "there is nothing physically wrong with you that we can find." Or worse: "It's just all in your head."

My life had become focused on when, where, and how the healing would start, and on my first grandchild's pending birth. Both had a parallel meaning—a new beginning.

My appointment with my immunologist finally arrived. I'd been waiting with bated breath in anticipation for a positive outcome in a direction of further healing and possibly remission.

I was more than ready. List in hand of point-blank questions and scientific articles and data to back up my quest, we made the three-hour drive to downtown Toronto. We knew the drive so well after doing the commute for years. The hospital's sterile environment had no effect on my senses, as I had become desensitized physiologically to my surroundings. I still was, however, reactive in adverse ways to the smells and lighting. I was, as usual, medicated to the max to go out into the regular world. My antihistamines were a lifesaver. My EpiPen was ready to go in my purse. Thankfully, I'd never had to use it, as it's the last line of defense for me having too much norepinephrine running in my bloodstream from dysautonomia and hyper-POTS. Zantac bottles jingled in my purse, even though I had taken myself off them seven months prior. Another emergency stash of Benadryl sloshed around in double Ziploc baggies. Liquid meds and an expensive Coach purse did not mix well. Once bitten, twice shy. I was more than ready for any emergency. I was ready for this outing.

My appointment went well, and we were moving forward in the quest to find antibodies. Only the immunologist wouldn't be doing the testing. He referred me back to my cardiologist. I reminded myself that I was being proactive as I messaged his assistant after a week-and-a-half wait to ensure she had received the referral to have the antibody testing done. I got a quick reply and an appointment six weeks away. *I can do this*, I told myself. Waiting six weeks was a piece of cake. One I couldn't eat, but a piece of cake nonetheless.

I told my closest friends and shared the thread of hope within our little family. It was positive, and I tried not to invest too much emotionally in the pending testing and the chance at treatment and remission. I tried to focus on the little bundle who would be arriving soon.

The day arrived sooner than expected. Not the specialist appointment, nope, I mean the BIG day. The life-changing day. The joyful day when our life would never again be the same, thank goodness! We got the call that our grandchild was on his way. We were over the moon with excitement. Nash Jeffery James made his entrance on April 20, 2018, at 3:51 p.m. I wept with joy but felt overwhelmed that I would miss out on so much of his future if I didn't get the appropriate treatment.

I had learned by deep gratitude and some practice to live in the moment. I took in his tiny fingers and toes. The breathtakingly beautiful features of this little man. My heart was bursting with happiness and much pride and love for the new parents. He was—and is—my joy!

One week after the elation of Nash's birth, my world came crashing down. Our beloved sixteen-year-old Yorkie, Abby, needed to be assisted in her passing. It's in those moments that we realize we are not "putting them down," but that our love and selfless act is raising them up out of pain and suffering. As positive as that sounds, my heart was broken into tiny pieces. We were at peace with the decision because we knew it was coming, and it was time. It was as if she held on long enough for my grandson to be born. It's as if she knew her exit strategy and that perhaps my heart would not break as much. She had been an active role in helping me cope with my illness. She always seemed to smell or sense when an attack was coming prior to its arrival. She gave me unconditional love, tons of laughter, comfort, and so much happiness! I will miss her more than words can say. My princess Abigail, gone forever, but forever in my heart.

My heart was torn to pieces, and I uttered the words over and over: Never again. Never again.

NEVER AGAIN!

NOTE TO SELF

In the moment of heartache and sorrow, it is okay to not be okay. It is also okay to recognize that statements that reflect not wanting to allow your heart to fill with joy, happiness, love, and purpose is an immediate solution for the inevitable passing of someone or something you once deeply loved. It is easier to build up walls than to work through the pain of heartache.

Building walls is not a journey but the extinguishing of feelings. Remember, when walls go up, they keep the bad feelings out, but more so, they impede the good feelings from getting in.

Remember, your motto: "I am more afraid of not feeling alive than I am of dying."

Feeling alive encompasses a cycle, allowing our heart to feel the depth of love and joy, and the depth of grief that sometimes follows, so we can feel gratitude and appreciation for the gift of repeating the cycle.

TAKE A MOMENT FOR YOURSELF

Breathe, Pause, Reflect . . .

Do you have walls or build walls? If so, is it more to protect your heart from people or animals?

Most will say people. If you said people, then who? This list of people allows you to recognize both the difference between building a wall and setting boundaries. Walls are not self-care, but healthy boundaries are.

Can you safely dismantle the walls and choose to place boundaries with those individuals in order to keep within your alignment?

Can you see how walls built keep out both bad and good feelings?

Walls are a type of detachment for all forms of emotions. They provide a false front that usually cannot be maintained (in a healthy individual). They eventually crumble for good reason. Setting healthy boundaries is the best approach.

Key to a Special Heart

I birthed a baby boy,
a miracle to this day.
I held him in my arms,
loving unconditionally, one would say.

I watched him grow to toddler,
then teen and then a man.
His heart I protected,
cherished and nurtured,
as his life began.

"Love you to the moon and back"
those words I'd love to say.
They still hold true for my sweet boy,
in every breath I say.

I would hold him tight,
my precious child.
His words loving and true.
"Mommy, when I grow big,
I'm going to marry you."

In those days I held
so very close from the start,
I held a special key,
a key for a special heart.

I knew this day would come,
and so I say to you.
I could not have picked a better
person, your love is oh so true.

May you always feel the special love
I felt right from the start.
I hand to you a special key,
a key for a special heart.

CHAPTER 21

HOPE

My appointment with the cardiologist was weeks away. As hard as I tried, I couldn't let go of the thread of hope, as it felt like that was all I had right then. The thoughts that I might be able to eat a variety of foods or even safely travel again were swirling in my brain. I was giddy with excitement and so optimistic and hopeful that I was talking openly about the future and looking online at recipes and trips. Then it occurred to me that I was setting myself up for disappointment. What if he didn't want to test me? What if he did, but the test came back negative? All hope would be exhausted, and I'd be right back in the same position I was in at that moment. The realization of that was numbing. It was more than I could bear.

The fear and doubt crept into my thoughts. The "what ifs" clouded my positivity. I had moments of tears and verbalized my fears of treatment and my fears of not getting treatment. My level of acceptance if the test was negative failed me. I would be crushed, devastated, and left with zero direction for an improvement in my health. The realization of that was so overwhelming that I tried my best to live in the moment. In that moment, I still had hope. In that moment, I loved and lived each day to the best of my ability, taking in every moment of joy I could. I filled my days with gratitude for everything I had and everything I could do instead of what I couldn't do. I had so much in life to be grateful for.

The day finally arrived. We were off for my appointment with my cardiologist. I was filled with anticipation over the latest development. I was filled with hope and promise that we were closing in on this elusive illness that had taken every essence of who I was.

The appointment started off on a different foot, and I insisted that Jeff come into the room to hear and see everything. He acknowledged my request and followed me into the examination room.

The appointment didn't go as expected. The specialist acknowledged that he hadn't seen me since 2015. (It was now May 2018.)

"Yes, I slipped through the cracks, as I have with various other specialists."

I waited for a reply to my comment. There was none.

We went through my symptoms and checked my blood pressure and heart rate, reclining and standing. All standard with a postural orthostatic tachycardia diagnosis.

The cardiologist indicated that I needed three medications to stabilize me. Both Jeff and I were a bit taken aback. I mentioned that the immunologist referred me back to him again specifically for antibody testing.

I made eye contact with him and said, "Check my file. I already have confirmed hyper-POTS. I want to be tested for antibodies."

"No," the doctor said. "We are not doing that. This is the medication you need. Your adrenergic number is too high. It should be a 3, maximum, and you have a confirmed blood draw of 8.9." His pointer finger hit the computer screen over and over as he spoke.

The antibodies test, discussion, and any hope were all shut down in a twenty-minute conversation. I left devastated, crushed, and hopeless. I held back tears, knowing that crying would create hives on my skin. I held back the lump in my throat, knowing the sobs that would follow, and I did my best to save Jeff both the embarrassment and the burden of dealing with me in such a state right there in the cardiologist's office.

We made our way to the parking garage, and I was shocked to silence for fear of the words that would escape my mouth. We'd barely driven out of the parking garage when the tears started. The sobbing followed.

The words finally slipped from my lips: "I don't want to do this anymore. I can't live with the pain, the symptoms, the psychological torture of not eating and having to go through life watching everyone around me eat. They enjoy life, they celebrate with food and wine and bond over them. I sit and watch the food go in their mouths, I smell it, I hear them chew."

All the foods I loved and the joy and comfort they brought to me were forever out of touch, gone like the strands of hope I clung to for the antibodies testing and treatment that would follow.

"It's like the cardiologist was just doing a first diagnosis. It felt off. It felt like I was a new patient being diagnosed. I was sent for testing. I wasn't being sent to get diagnosed all over again. It felt fucking off. It's like the cardiologist had never laid eyes on me before and I was a new patient. Something wasn't right about it, Jeff. I feel it in my gut."

"Well, I kept track of the time. We were barely in there twenty minutes. I thought it was fast and rushed, myself. Maybe we should get someone else, babe." Jeff's voice sounded defeated as well.

My waves of sobbing and talking came to an abrupt silence as I logically tried to get a grip on the numbers. I needed to focus on the numbers. Maybe the cardiologist was right in the fact that the 8.9 was nowhere close to 3.

Did I need medication to calm down that hyper-response? Yes.

Did it make sense to me that even if we did do the antibodies testing and it confirmed it, they could treat with IVIG? Yes.

The reality would still be that the high number would need to be addressed prior to anything else as my body would—as it has done with every other medication and food item put in my mouth—scream.

REJECT.

ABORT MISSION.

HOUSTON, WE HAVE A PROBLEM.

My logical/clinical brain was winning out in short order, and I calmly reached into my purse to pull out the prescriptions. The cardiologist was, in my mind, a brilliant doctor. The assessment had been accurate, as had the prescription of the medication to lower the 8.9 number to decrease hypersensitivity as well as control and balance blood flow and heart rate. It made sense. But still, my gut feeling of the appointment was off. Was it all in my head?

I glanced at the three prescriptions written on a single slip. I did my best to make out the handwriting and gave kudos to pharmacists everywhere, as they had to be experts in the gibberish that they often received. I was able to make out the medications prescribed and dose for each. For the first time ever, I was prescribed an antianxiety medication. Or so I thought. The reasoning was that I had too much adrenaline and norepinephrine. The same small dose at bedtime had been used with success for patients of MS, lupus, and seizures.

I found that interesting in a couple of ways. One, it was used and was successful for autoimmune patients. Second, the seizure/convulsion/storms aspect of my disease had been skirted over by just about every doctor. I labeled them as "attacks." This was the first time the formality of what they really were was briefly mentioned.

I would give it a go and maybe it would calm the storm before it started when trying something new. Usually, the cascade of symptoms that followed trying something new left me debilitated for weeks on end.

But my logical brain marked it up to losing credibility with anyone in the medical community. I needed to face them in the future and make them take me and my disease seriously. It also made me hesitant to discuss my medication with friends and family, as some would judge. Now, with this new medication, the focus would be on anxiety. I knew this fear was justified because it's a stigmatism that many individuals face.

Well, I already knew I had anxiety, mainly a slight social anxiety. My fear was that the illness would be overlooked and dismissed, and others would say, "See, it's just anxiety."

And those who say, "It's just anxiety" have never experienced anxiety. Their perspective is clouded with rose-colored glasses. Lucky buggers.

I have immense empathy for the double whammy of anxiety and depression. It's a bitch! It's a bastard! It's a beast to be tamed.

I would give the medications a gallant effort to get them in me.

As I was about to put the prescriptions back in my purse, I glanced at the top where my personal information should have been. My name wasn't on the prescription. My health card information wasn't on the sticker placed at the top by my cardiologist. A sense of panic overcame me as I read it again. I waved it to get Jeff's attention while he was driving. Not the best of ideas.

My venting poured out as I became overwhelmed with anger, frustration, and utter disbelief. I read some other patient's name, address, health card information, PCP information, and phone number off the top of the prescription. I was dumbfounded. We were one-quarter of the way home on our three-hour drive. I quickly grabbed my cell and called the cardiologist's office.

Voice mail.

"Nope, not good enough."

I tried again. Voice mail.

"Nope, not having this today."

I called the hospital's main number and requested to be directed to the cardio unit where the cardiologist was located. The receptionist picked up, and I immediately said that I'd just had an appointment with the doctor, and I was now one-quarter of the way home and the prescription slip had some other patient's information on it. I quickly read her the patient information before she put me on hold. She promptly came back on the line and asked if I could come back to the cardiac clinic.

Seriously? Would you want to go back? Would you feel like you would be composed to go do a face-to-face? I would lose my shit right there in front of everyone.

"Nope, not happening," I told the assistant. I said, "We traveled three hours to get there and have three hours to get home."

She put me on hold yet again. In anticipation, I pulled out a recent pill bottle that was filled at the new drug store close to our new condo that hadn't closed yet for the day. I knew she'd ask for my pharmacist's information to fax in the prescriptions. She returned and apologized for the delay and asked if I knew my pharmacist's info. She should have been relieved that I had it ready to go. Before she hung up, I asked for her name; she replied and assured me that she would fax it in right away.

My mind was now swirling with doubts and lack of confidence. Questions emerged. Did the doctor have the right file? Yes, I assured myself; I was called in by the shortened version of my name: Anne.

Was the doctor looking at my file on screen while pointing out the blood draw numbers?

Yes, I again assured myself. I knew those numbers. They were a validation to me in the past. A marker in testament that finally showed a valid scientific number to collaborate my illness. My head was spinning, as I was now feeling angry at this change in events. I was angry the antibody testing had been pushed aside and now even more angry that this error with the prescription had happened. Yet it ate at me that he dismissed me and tried to argue about my symptoms, a main one of which he said I have never had. He indicated that I did not need antibodies tested as I never had GI issues. That right there is when I should have abruptly spoken up and called him out on his error. I never got the opportunity, as he quickly dismissed us. My first symptom was GI issues. It was diagnosed as a virus. Then possibly flared IBS. Then possibly, who the hell can even remember? I'd honestly lost track. Sometimes I felt like I might as well have just put up a dart board and labeled each section with a diagnosis or potential. Here, grab a dart, give it a throw, and let's see what it potentially could have been that caused and is still causing the debilitating GI issues.

I DID NOT FEEL HEARD.

I DID NOT FEEL SEEN.

I DID NOT FEEL CONFIDENT IN THE CARDIOLOGIST.

I DID NOT FEEL I WANTED TO TRUST THOSE ERRORS WITH MY HEALTH, WITH MY LIFE.

I sat in silence the remainder of the drive home as I took it all in. The reality was that some of us would get lost in a sea of symptoms and a vast number of specialists, and some of us would fall through the cracks.

All of it nagged at me as I closed my eyes on a very long and emotionally disappointing day. My last thoughts before falling asleep were: *I can't do this anymore. I don't want to do this anymore.* The endless doctors' appointments and still no management. The searching for treatment so I could live a better quality of life was exhausting.

I heard all the doctors' words in my head, saying over and over: "This isn't going to go away. We need to manage it. It won't get any better." Yet, no one really has stepped up to manage it correctly.

I was a prisoner in my own body. One that has its own mind. I professed my love to Jeff and thanked him yet again for his support on this emotionally disappointing day for both of us. I turned away from him so he didn't see the tears roll down my cheeks. I held back the lump in my throat, wanting to escape in sobs. I buried my face into the pillow so he wouldn't hear the heart-wrenching cries. I had way too much practice at the art of muffling sobs.

My thoughts briefly went to my beloved Abby. We had made the difficult decision to assist with her passing five weeks prior. I missed her terribly, and in that moment, I felt a tinge of envy that she'd been allowed to escape her illness, relieved of having to struggle yet another day from a painful disease that would not go away.

I awoke early. My phone read 5:30 a.m. I couldn't sleep; my mind was just too busy. I rose and readied myself for my day of travel to visit the kids and our new grandson, Nash. I was looking forward to our visit. I felt excited, yet I knew gathering where there was food and wine was still a struggle. But I have always found the strength to push on, forward.

The time spent with the kids was a needed break from my reality. I got through another visit but struggled emotionally as they ate their steak with garlicky mushrooms swimming in butter and their Caesar salad, my favorite. In reality, I was grappling with my emotions from the previous day. I struggled to eat my potato soup and latkes. My head was down, and I was quiet during the conversation as the thoughts in my head went to how all hope was now gone. This was my life, and I didn't want to do this anymore. It was too emotionally painful. It wasn't that I wanted to take my life. What I wanted was a resolution, a plan, a treatment, and a management team so I could mainly eat without becoming violently ill and get assistance to live a normal life, a better quality of life. After all these years of living with chronic illness, I still feel the heavy weight of carrying that burden alone, of having the tenacity to remove myself from the cracks of what I believe is a broken medical system.

We left to head home, and I again pushed myself into silence, glancing at the landscape as we drove. The view was of deep, rich spring foliage and baby calves and colts frolicking in fields.

My phone chimed with emails and text messages and missed calls. I ignored all. I continued to take in the landscape as we passed farm after farm. I have always loved farms. It had been a dream to have a mini farm: a few chickens, a goat or two. A mini pony would be nice. We had the land for it. The pony would be a stretch. I could hear Jeff in my head. The work and commitment, with heavy emphasis on the work part. We were too soft. We had discussed it briefly in the past, but it went in different directions—mine naming the chickens Henrietta and Penelope, and other pairs of female names that brought a smile to my face: Lucy and Ethel or Thelma and Louise.

I remember Jeff laughing and saying, "How are you going to feel when winter comes, and we have to slaughter the birds to eat and get new ones in the spring?"

I was mortified. "Over my dead body," was my loud protest.

He laughed and said how he knew me too well, just imagining what our Christmas card photo would look like with our farm animals.

"So exactly what would that photo look like?"

"The fireplace is roaring. You and I are posed sitting on the floor, while the chickens, goats, mini pony, and the dogs sit on the sofa behind us."

We really had a good laugh about it all. I felt no shame in admitting his statement about the photo was both funny and true. We were too soft to be farmers, even on a mini scale.

I blinked back to my reality and realized we were five minutes from our lake house. When we arrived home, the silence between Jeff and me was typical; he knew to leave me to my thoughts or a good book or writing, and I left him to watch hockey.

My thoughts generally made it to my journal, notes, or laptop. I am a writer, and I always have been. I still remember the hard cardboard little plaid case with acrylic handle I once had. I kept all my secrets written down on lined paper. All my drawings, doodles, and snippets of childhood innocence were locked away in that case. The thought of that plaid case brought a smile to my face.

NOTE TO SELF

Hope is not lost. As long as I have a breath left in this body, I will hold hope in my heart.

It had been a bad few days. When I viewed them after "Breathe, Pause, Reflect . . . ," what I really felt was disappointment, disbelief, and sadness. I felt unheard and unseen, nothing more than a number. I felt dismissed. I felt gaslighted. I felt I was not being helped in any manner by the majority to develop a successful direction and a plan for management, so I could lead and have a better quality of life.

TAKE A MOMENT FOR YOURSELF

Breathe, Pause, Reflect . . .

Losing a beloved pet, a fur baby, is a loss like no other. For me, the mourning was horrible. Have I healed? At times I think I have. But there are days that I can't even mention Abby's name without tears. Grief is like that. It ebbs and flows.

Have you had a beloved fur baby who has passed?

Do you have wonderful memories that make you laugh, smile, and bring you joy?

Hold on to those. Those are the memories worth holding on to.

The Last Time

They will greet you at the door with pure joy and love,
you won't even know it was the last time.

They will give you love, joy, and tug at your heartstrings.
Lap it up, so to speak.

One day you will have a wonderful cuddle, a wet kiss,
and feel that unconditional love, and "it," my friends, will
be that last time, and you won't even know it.

That last time will sneak up on you.
In truth, most people don't even know that it's the last
time for anything.
So, make those moments count, as it might just be that
last time.

CHAPTER 22

THE UNDERDOG

2019

Well, if you are not by now cheering for the underdog, the warrior who lives another day to have longer breaths between battles, you really should be. I happened to play for the Invisible Team of Chronically Ill, a team, sadly, that's immensely large. If you can't see us, then brace yourself, we are about to get loud. Really, really loud—so we can All Be Heard!

I gather you might be saying . . .

Oh, please let this have a happy ending!

Please let it all end well!

I say . . .

Cheer for the underdog, the warrior. I am not a betting woman, but I would bet on me.

I would bet that I will . . .

Never give up!

Not on myself, my children, my grandchildren, and other relationships that mutually nurture.

I will never quit trying . . .

To do better and to be a better person than I was the day before.

I will always practice self-care and make my health, body, and mind a priority.

Nothing is more important than your health, physically and mentally. Nothing—and I mean nothing!

So many things come to light when you are chronically ill. All that time spent working and trying to strive for a larger income to pay for a larger house, car, trips, educations. So many hours spent being busy, too busy. My prized purses, shoes, and power suits had little meaning as I lay chronically ill in a bed for more than a year during 2012 and part of 2013. I could not wear the heels and had no need to have a purse that matched. All the rushing and planning and taking care of everyone. Being the rock to many through divorces, breakups, health scares, family and money issues meant I rarely took time for myself.

I didn't invest in my own health in a committed way. It just wasn't a priority. I didn't view myself as a priority because everyone else always came first. I was already burned out to a degree prior to my sister Nancy's illness. Her passing should have been my wake-up call to make myself a priority. I didn't hear the universe whisper; or did I just ignore it? The universe had to throw a brick at me to notice that changes needed to happen.

By 2019 so much had changed. There is always a new normal when you have pivotal moments. They get labeled as "pre-kids," "pre-divorce," "pre-trauma," "pre-illness." They are generally the "prequel" of life's journey as we look back in hindsight. I sat in my newly found vintage midcentury modern chair and my mind went back a few years to the day I messaged my goddaughter KK to come and get her pick of my shoes. My sadness at losing the ability to wear heels due to mobility issues was replaced by the joy of her smile when she thanked me for the endless boxes of shoes.

I was at a standstill once again. I felt discouraged and didn't know what to do, as trying any new food upset my immune system to attack with vengeance. But was I really at a standstill?

I paused and looked out at the lake as its water ripples crested the rocky point. I stood on my yoga mat and stretched my hands overhead. I bent down and touched my toes. I moved to the mat and sat in lotus pose and breathed. I took in my breath. In, hold; out, hold; in, hold; out, hold.

In that moment, it was as if I had just suddenly woken up to realize how far I had come over the time since we moved to the lake. It was as if I'd forgotten how far I'd come from being bedridden. Not forgotten—more like I just didn't want to remember. But I did remember it, all too well.

It'd almost been a year since my last attack. I know, however, that the attacks were part and parcel of my type of dysautonomia, a disorder of the autonomic nervous system (ANS). The attacks were actually "storms." They were norepinephrine and cytokine in nature, causing a symptom of seizure-like convulsions.

There, I said it. I put it out there. Does it sound a lot worse than it is? I can assure you, unfortunately, it was—and is—that bad. I did, however, at that moment in time, focus on the fact they had subsided tremendously.

Why? What was the change? Why and how did the transformation happen?

How in the hell could I even allow my internal narrative to feel disappointed or judge how far I had come? Things have changed in many areas of my life. I have changed them to transition into the new pivot of life.

Why?

The question was more a "how" than anything else.

I stopped asking the "why" in life quite a few years back. I no longer looked desperately for what caused my chronic illness. It no longer mattered. I was confident, as were most specialists, that it was, in fact, viral overload.

When I first became ill, the majority of doctors gave the same bleak outcome of perhaps this was as good as it was going to get. I was bedridden at the time. There was no cure. This was the best we could all do.

I refused to believe it. I chose to believe in the body's ability to heal itself to a degree. To repair the damage done. I chose to work with that, rather than throw in the towel and say it wouldn't get any better than being bedridden.

Had I traveled a rough journey to get to where I was now? One hundred percent.

But look where I was now. Look how far I had come. I had so much to be and feel grateful for. The simple things that most take for granted: bathing and washing my own hair. Walking, and not just to get from the bed to the bathroom, the route I used to crawl. Now, I was outright walking, in minus twenty-five-degree weather, doing between three and five kilometers per day. Holy shit! How did that happen?

By summer of 2019, I was helping on the property, and it was damn hot out, sweltering, in fact.

I was working away, but then I noticed dribbles down my inner thighs.

"Shit. Oh, my God, I think I just peed myself." There was a look of horror on my face.

"What?" Jeff looked at me in disbelief.

I pointed to my legs. Then I noticed my back felt very wet.

"Babe, you're sweating! Holy shit, babe, you are sweating. Do you feel okay? Maybe I should get you some water to keep hydrated."

Yep, I was sweating, like a normal person. Jeff and I were both so shocked. Sweat was running off my back and down my legs. You've never seen two happier people over seeing the sweaty wet marks on my T-shirt, like the proof of a miracle. We cheered our bottles of water as we found so much happiness and gratitude in that simple, normal bodily function.

The simple things that most individuals take for granted. That's not a jab at anyone. I was one of those individuals—until I wasn't.

I had to really pause and dig deep into the road of healing. I had to backtrack to see when it actually started. How did it start? What did I do to get to where I was now?

Was the path to healing linear? Cough . . . news alert . . . linear is straight. Linear involves proportional changes. Linear is a forward progression in stages equal and sequential.

Life and healing are not linear!

So, I went to work. I set out on a new path of writing, one that took all the fragmented pieces and placed them together so I could see the puzzle of healing.

I pulled together all the details of my life over the last number of years, even some that looked to be irrelevant. In reality, they were all steps in the healing process.

A simple thing for me to remember was that "less is more."

I had to dig even deeper to acknowledge and notate the changes I had made.

The courses, education, and practices I had taken.

I obtained my re-certification as a Certified Coach Practitioner.

I obtained certificates in Applied Polyvagal Theory and enriched my mind with Integrative Trauma Therapy. I expanded my area of practice in breath work and cryotherapy, meditation, and yoga.

I did so, as I was investing in myself. Fully investing in myself in all practices to heal.

There were additional benefits.

The individuals I had met along my journey and that nurtured my soul.

The lifestyle changes I made.

How did the healing happen? That is a rhetorical question. I know how healing happened!

NOTE TO SELF

The unknown is sometimes scary. Remaining in the same painful state is terrifying. Sometimes you need to step out of your comfort zone and take educated risks. Healing is a journey, but it is not linear. Learn to congratulate yourself along the way. The baby steps count. The steps back count, if only for the fact you are still willing to take another in the direction forward with an open mind and an open heart. No one is going to take the first steps for you.

NOTE TO YOU

You must continue to choose you, yourself. You have already started—you're reading this book. Congratulations. Continue to educate yourself in what your body and mind need. If you need help with direction, that's what I am here for. You are not alone in this battle.

You are thinking to yourself, "Yeah, sure, she's an author. She won't respond if I reach out."

I bet you I will respond.

TAKE A MOMENT FOR YOURSELF

Breathe, Pause, Reflect . . .

It is so clear when I stop and think about it. When I breathe, pause, and reflect.

I really took steps forward in healing. Sometimes in leaps and bounds. But part of me wasn't ready to embrace gratitude, fully. There was still this expectation of getting my life back fully and completely to the way it had been. I had not reached full acknowledgment of the fact that life was never going to be exactly the same again. When you go through a full-blown catastrophic storm, you don't emerge unscathed on the other side of it. Acknowledging your physical and mental traumas is half the battle to healing. Perhaps trying to be the person you were "before" delays healing. That person, on some levels, does not exist in the present moment. Acceptance and gratitude are growth in knowing you have come a long way. Breathe as if your life depended on giving breath to that person.

Life is a journey.

Can you think of issues or pivots in the past that you've battled through?

Did you or have you given yourself credit for having the strength required to succeed?

Sometimes the little things really matter. Baby steps really matter.

Each day that you take a positive step forward in life, breathe, pause, reflect, and congratulate yourself.

CHAPTER 23

ACT III—LOOKING FORWARD

How did I get here? How did this actually happen? The journey seemed so impossible at times. I was upended and shaken to the core. That is saying it mildly. I am just going to be authentically me here and call a spade a spade.

I'm going to be brutally honest and honestly brutal. It was a new level of hell on earth. It sucked the life out of me. Mind, body, and soul.

I have put together a list of the areas of life that I felt were a key factor in my healing. I am not a doctor. I can only state what has worked for me and others in their own healing journey. I am a life coach who specializes in chronic health and trauma. I also work with adoptees or individuals looking for family. Again, both have waves of trauma with a root cause, be it a health root or a family tree root.

HEALTH ADVOCACY

One of the hardest things I had to learn about this journey was that no one is going to rush to save you. No one is going to make your health their priority.

You have to save your damn self! You have to make yourself a priority, mentally, physically, and peacefully.

I now come first. Not because I am better than anyone else. I come first for the choices and decisions I make for my mental and physical well-being. My health is my priority—it's as simple as that!

Being your own health advocate is key. If you cannot, then work to find someone who can assist you to be your advocate in the manner that works for you both.

KEY COMPONENTS FOR A SUCCESSFUL HEALTH ADVOCATE

Communication skills to provide calm, clear explanations of your health concerns and requirements are needed. Provide information regarding your medical history. A permission letter will be required to discuss your information with any healthcare provider. It also gives a clear mutual direction of communication between your health advocate and your health provider.

Choosing an individual you trust who can maintain discretion and is understanding and caring is highly recommended.

A strong health advocate should have the traits of being assertive, organized, and confident in asking questions and in advocating for you. They need calm, clear, and direct communication skills.

I am my own health advocate, as are many others. It is estimated that approximately 70 percent of individuals are their own health advocates.

So, I will repeat one of my family's favorite movie quotes from *The Godfather*, used in one of my favorite movies, *You've Got Mail*: "Go to the mattresses."

It's a battle. Be your own health advocate. No one is going to do it for you!

MENTAL HEALTH

My personal thoughts are that there is no way to healing without a mental health cycle going through the stages. I want everyone, healthy and chronically ill individuals, to know that from my perspective, becoming chronically ill is a loss of oneself. It can cause the same cycle of grieving as the loss of someone you love. After all, when you're chronically ill, you're grieving the loss of your healthy life, the loss of yourself, prior to chronic illness.

Anyone who knows even a little bit about grief knows it's a process that you work through. And it has stages, but not all stages are equal. Sometimes you can bounce back a stage or two as you work through the process. The one thing I have learned about grief is that there is no time limit. Grief is unique to each person, just as each person is unique.

Grief has no boundaries. You can grieve losing someone. You can grieve losing a fur baby. You can grieve losing yourself. I wish more people would look at chronic illness and recognize that it is truly and honestly a grieving process. Losing yourself and the life you have created and all your plans for your future often get washed away into the depths of the disease and all the struggles that go with it.

I once remarked to someone struggling with their own journey that grief can be like a sunny day. I watched her perplexed face in the Zoom meeting. She tilted her face from shoulder to shoulder as she tried to wrap her mind around my words as I explained, "Grief is like the sun on a beautiful, bright sunny day. You are driving down a country road, glancing at the stunning fields of green. The trees blow in the slight breeze. The windows are open, and the fresh air feels magnificent. The radio plays a song that makes you feel emotional. You crest the bend and turn up onto a hill where you are met with burning sunlight, blocking out your view. It's blinding; you can't see a thing. Instinctively, you slow down. Taking your foot off the gas, you almost stop, but you keep going slowly until the sun no longer blinds your eyes. The important thing is that you slowed down, took your time, did it your way. Grief is like the blazing sun. It can blind you, catch you off guard. The importance is that you keep moving forward."

Based on the Kübler-Ross Grief Cycle, there are five stages of grief

Denial:
Avoidance, confusion, elation, shock, fear.

Anger:
Frustration, irritation, anxiety.

Bargaining:
Struggling to find meaning, reaching out to others, telling one's journey, outright bargaining with the universe, God, faith.

Anyone who knows me will tell you flat out that I'm not a religious person, but I am spiritual in my own way. But boy, did I try to negotiate, bargain, and beg. Can I say that I prayed? Well, I did get on my knees and plead, making unrealistic exclamations and offering up all sorts of bargains with my hands pressed together and my eyes looking up in search for someone, anyone, to listen and to help.

I think that anytime you are truly in an emotional and physical crisis, you go wherever you feel you can to find an ounce of hope. Will this journey test even the most devout individuals? Yes, I think it will.

That was the beginning of negotiating with myself to move my life's journey forward. To put one foot in front of the other, I needed to bargain my way there. At times, it was like trying to negotiate with a toddler: "If you take one more bite of food and don't throw it up, you can watch another hour of TV."

I spent the next part of my journey making bargains that would never be fulfilled. Trust me, skip the bargaining stage, if you can. Grasp onto hope, peace, and positivity. That will help you jump further ahead in the stages of the journey.

Depression:

Feeling overwhelmed and helpless.

Did I fall in and out of depression? I would be lying to you if I said no. Depression is an old, haggard friend. I suffered post-partum depression for a year and a half after the loss of our girls, then after the birth of our third son, who is now twenty-nine years old. It's one of those things that Jeff and I look back on and say, "Ah, that seems so obvious now." People didn't really talk about postpartum depression thirty years ago. I now recognize the signs as I wavered in and out of feeling down, low, and downright depressed since becoming chronically ill.

I did go to therapy, and it did help me with coping skills that had gone to the wayside, so new ones needed to be developed. I learned so much about myself, of who I was prior to post-viral. How I used food, shopping, and wine to a degree to cope with several areas in my life, mainly stress and emotions. It took me awhile to recognize that anger is not the first response. Meaning, if you feel anger, there always is an emotion that comes before it. Learning this and becoming aware of it was key. When I'm feeling angry, I now pause to honestly reflect on what triggered the anger. Digging deep is essential to healing emotionally. When you do so, sometimes you uncover deep-rooted wounds that have never healed. It made some relationships even more complex. There were—and to a point, there still are—a lot of people in my life who want and need me to be who I was prior to my illness. I am not that person anymore.

I'm disappointed in others who haven't been who I needed and wanted them to be through this journey, and through my life, for that matter. If you emerge from a battle without a scar, then you are not human. To emerge with wounds that you work to heal and move forward with in your journey makes you a superhero in my eyes. I still work hard every day to be my own superhero. I work daily to be better all-around than I was the day before. I congratulate and give myself pep talks throughout my day as I embark on the next stage of my journey.

Acceptance:

Moving on, making the pivot, putting one foot in front of another in a forward direction, exploring options.

As you read through my journey, you will have picked up on some of my denial, anger, bargaining, depression, and finally, acceptance.

Acceptance is not throwing in the towel. Acceptance is making some decisions in your life for the moment. It is also accepting that you did the best you could with the options you had at a given moment in time.

I honestly do not know the exact day it happened. I guess it happens when you are ready for it. It isn't something you can force. It seemed to me like a natural progression, a transition. Looking back, I would have to say that the longer you fight it (acceptance to whatever part of your life or journey you need to personally accept), the harder the pivot will be.

It's a process. Some points of acceptance came quickly, but there were others I dragged out painfully, almost to the point of self-flagellating, as if getting sick wasn't punishment enough.

I remember the day I finally accepted that my career was over. In reality, it was over by the time I was well into my first year of being sick, and the bank knew that. But for me, it took being fired and having all my office items delivered to my home by courier. It took formal papers that needed to be signed and authenticated. It took packing up my diplomas and mementos into boxes and purging other meaningless objects. Acceptance came with the purging to release the invisible twine that kept me tethered to that part of my life that no longer served me.

I thought I would cry as I watched the garbage truck, then the recycling truck take away chunks of my long career. I felt a sense of fear of the unknown and freedom, all at the same time. I had done enough crying over my lost career. I had moved past it, moved forward, and fully accepted the change. That tears did not fall was a positive sign that I had turned a corner in my life, grown from the experience of having it and letting it go. That part of my life no longer served me, and I no longer served it.

Acceptance can encompass many aspects of your life as you strive forward through your journey.

Remember that healing is not linear. Grief ebbs and flows. There is no end to grief. It's more of a weighted scale that eventually becomes heavily weighted in acceptance and gratitude. Building up coping skills to manage the triggers so the pivot forward is more successfully managed is key.

If you have difficulty in walking through the cycles of grief and struggle with coping skills, then I highly recommend you find a qualified individual who can assist you.

Oh, the things some people say. When you are chronically ill and are struggling, it's important to have people around you who are understanding, kind, nurturing, and respectful.

There is a key difference in individuals who hurt your feelings.

Take a step back and see that their comments, although somewhat inconsiderate, were probably not said with intent to hurt. I have had people close to me say the damnedest things. When talking about someone else, they've said, "Nobody likes to be around a Debbie Downer; it's depressing."

Hearing that makes it difficult to trust and share your struggles. I've had someone say to me, "You can't eat; you can't drink. What in the hell am I supposed to do with you?"

Someone else said, "I miss the old Anne Marie. You know, the one who could eat and drink and was fun."

Other hurtful things said to me were:

"You look bloated. Maybe you should lose some weight. It will make you feel better about yourself."

"You look too thin. Maybe you should gain some weight. It will make you feel better about yourself."

This is not the story of *Goldilocks and the Three Bears*: you're too big; you're too small; now, you're just right. Let me fill you in on something—people who comment on your weight when you are chronically ill are not being kind. If the focus is on a superficial thought that you will feel better about yourself, they have lost the fact that you are chronically ill. I wanted to feel better as in healthier.

Unfortunately, all the hurtful reactions are hazards of having an invisible illness.

Those unkind statements are not outright attacks. Usually,

those statements are from individuals expressing the fact that they also miss the healthy person they knew before chronic illness. Were they thoughtful in using those words? No. But was it said to hurt me on purpose? No.

Unfortunately, there will also be some people in your life who have an agenda. They have a purpose and an intent with their meanness. They are the ones who attack, who manipulate, and who fill your life with chaos, stress, and drama. Beware of them.

Part of caring for your mental health is taking the steps to respect yourself enough to place boundaries that are for your wellness. It's a simple as that. The extent of the boundaries needed will vary from person to person. Creating a peaceful environment requires an act of purging on many levels. I say, "If it costs me my peace, it's too expensive!"

Additional activities assist with good mental health, like finding enjoyment in a hobby or creative projects. For me, it was writing, art, photography, and other small projects. And music, the kind that makes you want to dance. For me, it was a combination of the greatest hits of the '40s and the '70s. Creating a space that promotes joy, light, and vision doesn't just mean in your surroundings, it is also in your mind. You know what they say, "Music soothes the soul" and "Music soothes the savage beast." Think of the soul and beast being one of the same, the vagus nerve.

MINDSET

Pivoting with grace isn't the easiest of things to do when the direction of the pivot is completely and utterly unplanned. If the pivot is earth shattering and goes against the grain of your soul, we have no choices sometimes. I wish I could go back and tell myself, "Don't bloody well fight the pivot. Fight the disease, yes, but the pivot, no."

You reach a point when you realize in your mind that there is no going back to life before (blank). Go ahead and fill in your blank.

For me, it was chronic illness. There was no going back to life before chronic illness!

Sometimes you have to let go of the expectations, the image of how your life was going to turn out. Part of letting those expectations go is to learn to find joy in your journey at this moment in time. But joy is a tricky thing. The mind plays "remember when" a lot throughout the journey. For me, there was a lot of remembering all the things that brought me joy that I could no longer do. I had to LEARN to find the joy once more, in new things and in new ways. I found new hobbies, new passions, created new projects, and met many wonderful new individuals along this new part of my journey. Learning to let go and learning to find the joy in my journey was part of my healing.

Your mind knows you are making that pivot, but the heart, oh, it holds out as long as it can. I wish my heart would have listened to my mind. Frankly, it would have saved me a whole lot of heartache. Oh, trust me, it would have been like ripping off the Band-Aid. I say that, but I know my heart wasn't quite ready for it. I needed to learn so much from the journey. I took the long route.

Mindset is the key to happiness. Happiness and joyfulness are like food for the soul—food for the soul that brings you peace. And remember, whatever costs me my peace is too expensive.

I have chosen very carefully what I allow into my peaceful space. To heal the body and brain, I need a calm, peaceful environment.

I purged and set boundaries with those who did not mesh well with my healing and where my life was going. I chose to spend more time with individuals who fit my direction of journey, my future, not my history.

I also learned to edit my internal and external narrative. Creating a positive narrative takes work, especially when you are not feeling very positive.

I found the first steps of creating a daily positive journal cathartic.

Find yourself a small workbook or journal. The first page or two is dedicated to You! Write the numbers 1 to 100, leaving enough room for a single word to follow each number. Now, write a positive word that describes you next to each number. I know to some this sounds like a silly task and you're wondering what's the purpose?

The purpose is key. You are more than the disease, the illness, the whatever your (blank) was. You are so much more than that!

Once you have accomplished the 100, choose a time of day to journal. I like to journal right before I sleep. It pays to go to sleep on positive thoughts.

Some days, I write wonderful, lengthy, positive thoughts of the day. Other days, well, the sun was out, and I was breathing. The point I am trying to make is that there will be good and bad days. Even on the bad days, I could still find a hint of something to feel positive about.

We all become challenged when life throws us a monkey wrench. Take a deep breath and accept that there are things we absolutely cannot control. Moving to acceptance is both a challenge and a moment of calm. In reality, the only thing we can control is our attitude on this journey. It is a moment in time, and this too shall pass. It might as well pass with our best foot forward. It may propel us toward growth, understanding, empathy, and healing.

GROUPS

Oh, you know the groups I'm talking about here, the ones on social media. There are good groups and bad groups.

Don't get me wrong: I think if you're lucky enough to find a group that has an open administrator and allows open engagement with zero bullying, then fantastic! I really enjoyed some of the groups I was a part of. I felt the support there that I wasn't getting anywhere else. I felt heard, validated, understood. Some groups give wonderful support with scientific information, files, and articles, and they can be a great source for building your health advocacy attitude.

But if you find your enjoyment of the groups stops, if you feel that all the posts are making you feel down or you really wish someone would post more positive things, then it's time. It's time to readjust how often you keep in touch with the groups. I changed my notifications and only popped in when I wanted to see how things were going within the group. When I say, "it's time," I mean you are already making that pivot. Your brain is recognizing that it needs a more positive narrative. It's time!

VAGUS NERVE

The vagus nerve is a fundamental component of life and healing. The vagus nerve is actually made up of ten pairs of cranial nerves that supply and bring messaging for the function of the heart, lungs, the upper digestive GI tract, and additional functional organs of the chest and abdomen. The key aspect is that it innervates both the stomach and lungs.

The word "vagus" in Latin is well chosen; it literally means "wandering."

From my own personal journey, it is the key to healing and to the unlocking of understanding its function to implementing strategies to promote vagal tone.

Vagal tone = healing

Viral/bacterial/trauma = vagal dysfunction = chronic illness and trauma

When the vagus nerve functions at optimal levels, it systematically fires off appropriate signals to the cholinergic, anti-inflammatory pathway. In short, it's the gatekeeper to keeping the immune system running correctly.

The two primary organs of the immune system are the spleen and thymus. The vagus is the gatekeeper relaying information back and forth.

The thymus is the little warrior of the immune system. It destroys invaders that potentially cause threat. The thymus is, on average, fully functioning in size by puberty. After that stage, there is a decrease in size and function as we age. There are several factors that accelerate deactivation by hyper-stimulation of the organ such as virus and bacterial invaders, as well as high levels of stress and trauma. This deactivation puts us at a higher level of risk to chronic illness.

The spleen is the quality control keeper of the cells of the immune system. Its function is to weed out working and non-working cells of the immune system to promote the highest level of functionality. In short, chronic stress and trauma hinders the spleen's function, as does hyper-activation of the immune system when it becomes overwhelmed. The vagus nerve keeps the checks and balances of the parasympathetic and sympathetic activities for many organs. Overstimulation or hyper-stimulation decreases the spleen's functional abilities in properly targeting invaders by releasing an immune response of cytokines proteins to sound the alarm to the vagus nerve that relays the flags to the brain about the type of inflammation.

Strong vagal tone = health and healing

Increasing vagal tone can be achieved by several practices:

- Breathing exercises (see breath work)
- Gargling
- Activating the gag reflex
- Chanting or humming the "Om" used in the practice of Nāda yoga
- Cold exposure, such as cold showers, splashing cold water on your face, or ice plunges. (Caution needs to be taken if you are taking ice baths or icy lake plunges.)
- Side sleeping (I can attest to this one being 100 percent effective for me). I have confirmed postural orthostatic tachycardia (hyper-POTS). When I wake with a tachycardia episode, I shift to my left side and commence some deep breathing exercises (diaphragmatic breathing). My heart rate variability (HRV) shows significant reduction in tachycardia. Sleeping on my side and proper breath work

increases vagal tone. It assists in the reset of the vagus nerve to send proper signals to the autonomic nervous system. A study done by Yang et al. and published in the *Circulation Journal* confirms my personal findings are not just a random occurrence.

- Adopt patterns that promote restful sleep, such as decreasing stimulating hobbies like TV and all blue light electronics. Also, set a cutoff time of food and drink that works for you and your schedule.
- Last but not least, create a space of calm, of peace. For me, it's imperative that my space is clean, organized, and uncluttered (again, less is more). A clean and organized space promotes positive thoughts and a relaxed state of mind. Remove chaos from your space = chaos removed from your thoughts. Out of sight is often out of mind.

There's a reason people say to listen to your gut. Studies show that your gut (a.k.a. your digestive tract) has a vast amount of vagus nerve endings in the lining. It is a cholinergic anti-inflammatory pathway by way of neurotransmitters ACh.

The pathway of ACh is meant to relay signals to decrease inflammation and calm the immune system, but when we have invaders of the gut, the messages go out to the sympathetic nerves signaling a "flight or fight" response, releasing adrenaline and norepinephrine.

The gut and its microbial information relay the balance of secretions to both the sympathetic and parasympathetic nervous systems. It is what I call the "switch." When all is balanced, the switch turns on and off effortlessly. Unbalanced, it turns off and has difficultly turning on, or it turns on and has difficulty turning off. An example would be a hyper-response when the "fight or flight" is turned on and remains on high alert.

Highlight Cytokines (Release)

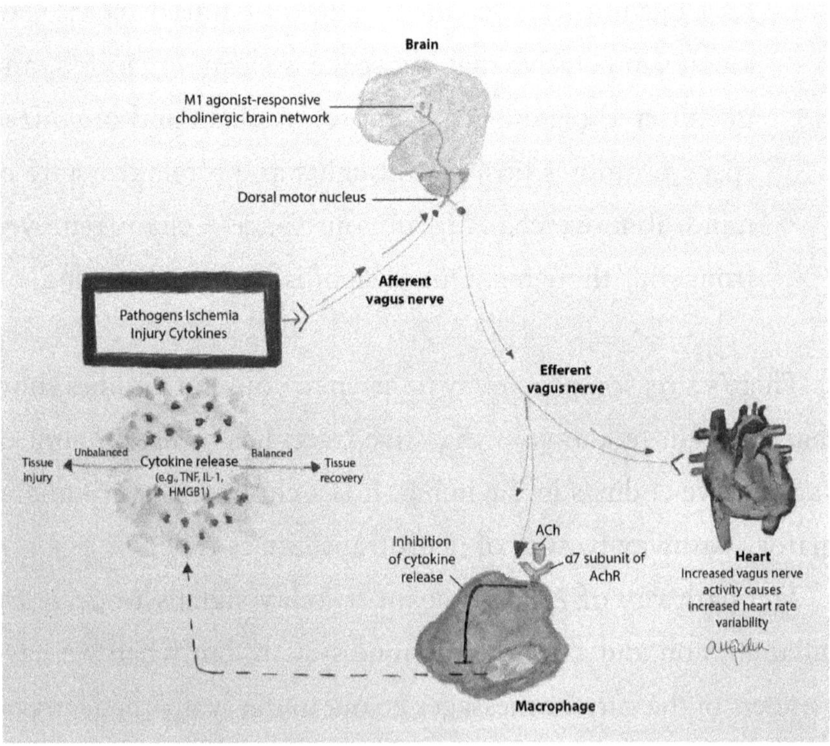

A cytokine release is a form of systemic inflammatory response syndrome that is triggered by a number of factors, including infection (viral and/or bacterial) or specific drugs/medications.

This systemic response causes a cytokine storm when a vast amount of white blood cells are activated and they then release inflammatory cytokine, which starts a cascade of additional white blood cells to be released.

Cytokine storms have been noted in long haul COVID-19 cases, as is with other diseases that cause a vast amount of systemic inflammatory response.

A cytokine storm is, in short, a hyperactive immune response and is mainly characterized by the release of chemokines or chemotactic cytokines (a family of small secreted proteins that signal protein receptors), interferons, interleukins, tumor-necrosis factors, and several other mediators. As a normal, healthy function, cytokines are imperative to effectively rid the body of the enemy of infectious agents. When cytokines go rogue, as in a cytokine storm, the huge levels of mediators are extremely detrimental to host cells.

I feel confident that in the near future, biomarkers will be confirmed to show a mixed autoinflammatory/autoimmune condition for dysautonomia and mast cell activation. In doing so, the expression of platelets being compromised by chronic inflammation. Blood panels will more likely involve testing several interleukin panels to support a dual inflammatory/autoimmune disease. I will continue to pursue this area of healing and will highlight articles, vetted research, and my own path progress and experiences on my website and on my private business profiles on social media. You can find more at www.amgodin.com.

DIET

As a noun, diet means the kinds of food habitually eaten (or avoided). As a verb, diet means a restriction of food eaten (often to lose weight). To avoid any confusion, I'm going to use the word fuel (diet as a noun).

I am not going to tell you the type of fuel you need to put into your body to make it run at an optimal level. There are a lot of issues with diet surrounding chronically ill individuals, including for myself. I am restricted to foods that do not set off a cascade of physical reactions within my body.

I will just keep it simple: Keep it lean, green, and clean. It's that simple.

Less is more. Less processed foods, fewer additives, more healthy choices.

When your gut produces an overgrowth of bacteria because of the wrong food choice and invaders, it causes a cascade of inflammation and toxins that eventually break down the barriers and enter the bloodstream.

Proper gut microbiome makes for a better information highway to the vagus nerve to relay the information to the brain.

For me, food has been an issue because I have mast cell and dysautonomia. Trying to take in medication and supplements has been better received via sublingual (under my tongue). Getting in the proper supplements and fluids fuels my body to aid in the process of breaking down and processing food items.

In this area, I had to ask a few things. Why sublingual? If the disease was truly an autoimmune disease, then why was there a difference in how I responded to something as simple as how vitamin B entered my body? For example, I can't take vitamin B in pill form, yet I can tolerate it by injection. I can't take a tablet form of Lorazepam, yet I can tolerate it sublingual.

The foods I can tolerate mostly all fall into the category of "high resistant starch" foods. These types of foods help feed the good bacteria growth in the gut by increasing short-chain fatty acids, most importantly butyrate. (Butyrate is a preferred energy source of your colon cells, reducing the pH and inflammation; it also reduces chances of developing colorectal cancer.) Also, this high resistant starch makes the food function as a soluble, fermentable fiber. These food items go through the stomach and the small intestine undigested, reaching the colon eventually to aid your friendly gut bacteria. I can only tolerate organic dark chocolate, 70 percent or higher, and only specific brands. Why? Roasted cocoa powder has a higher rate of butyrate and anti-oxidant properties.

Knowing all this information poses several questions:

1. Did the original viral cause damage to the gut, and is it reparable? In my case, I feel that the viral caused damage first to the gut, then the decline continued in the gut, setting as a catalyst to pathways/receptors in the messaging system via the vagus nerve and autonomic nerve system.
2. Could this be the same for the COVID long haulers? After all, a very high percentage of those patients fall under the chronic illness category of autonomic nerve dysfunction, dysautonomia, hyperimmune response, mast cell activation, and chronic fatigue.
3. Is fixing the brain and gut microbe axis part of the answer? Perhaps looking closer at the gut and mainly an unbalanced gut microbiome is more critical than many think. There is an article on healthline.com that quotes Dr. Ghannoum, Professor of Dermatology and Pathology at Case Western University School of Medicine, stating new studies have shown marked changes of the microbiome could affect how we respond to long-term COVID (after COVID-19). The study indicates that when dysbiosis has occurred, those after COVID-19 have higher symptoms. In fact, there were higher levels of unfriendly bacteria in individuals who showed long haul symptoms. The study linked some symptoms to specific unfriendly bacteria species.

This area of study intrigues me, as I have long thought prior to COVID-19 that fixing the gut to formulate a balanced microbiome aids the vagus nerve, which aids in healing. It has helped significantly when I changed my diet to remove gluten, particularly when it related to inflammatory pain.

I can't help but feel there will be great progress in this area in the future that could open many doors related to the brain and gut microbe axis and the immune system, healing, and mental health. I will continue to pursue this area of healing and will highlight articles, vetted research, and my own path progress and experiences on my website and on my private business profiles on social media. You can find more at www.amgodin.com.

MEDITATION

The act of meditating for mindfulness allows the body to go into a calm and meditative state, producing a positive response in your entire body and mind.

The benefits far outweigh the time it takes to put it into a practice. Those who say, "I don't have the time or the patience to meditate," need it even more.

Make the time. Think of it like brushing your teeth, something important that you need to do regularly. Your body and your mind will thank you.

Meditating helps reduce stress and improve coping skills for stress and triggers. It increases one's ability to be self-aware and to focus on the present. It can also reduce negative emotions and increase creativity, imagination, patience, and tolerance.

BREATH WORK

There are several breathing methods and techniques that can be practiced for better health, healing, and stress relief. You can start off with a smaller time span and eventually build to a longer duration. A good place to start is with a two- to five-minute practice, two or three times per day. I find it helps to keep track of my duration in time and sessions, and I use my phone timer and calendar to do that.

There are various techniques, although most share commonalities; I utilize several in my practice. To begin, get comfortable with breathing in your space by sitting or lying down. Be aware of your breath. Breath work is a practice best done as a daily routine, as well as whenever you feel necessary. I'll focus on breath work if I'm having a stressful day or feeling jittery.

Both inhale and exhale are equally important, as you breathe in oxygen and breathe out carbon dioxide. The breath in should feel natural, while the breath out should be extended and feel slightly forced.

First off, let's do a breathing test.

Lie flat on the floor. Place your right hand on your belly and your left hand on your chest.

Pay close attention to which hand rises first. Take in a full breath, hold to a count of four, and exhale.

Which hand rose first upon inhale? If you said the right hand on your belly, the breath was correct. If the left hand rose on your chest, there is work to do. It's simple work, but you have to retrain yourself to breathe properly, deeply.

BREATHING TECHNIQUES

Breath Focus:

A wonderful relaxation breathing technique to aid with calming.

You choose a mantra that works for you. It can be as simple as saying a word in your head as you inhale. For example: Peace (inhale); calm (exhale).

Give image to the inhale, bringing peace and calm, and the exhale, expelling any anxiety and tensions. Each exhale should be extended.

Inhale for a count of four, exhale for a count of eight, and finish with a sigh.

Repeat in a natural rhythm. Notice your face, neck, and shoulders for any form of tension. Release and continue your breathing practice.

Various other breathing techniques are:

Pursed/Pinched/Whistle Lip Breathing

Alternative Nostril Pressure/Nadi Shodhana
Equal Breathing Practice
Resonant/Coherent Breathing
Lion's Breath
Deep Breathing
Bee or Humming Breath
Sitali Breath
Breath of Fire
Belly/Diaphragm

Of all, I've found Belly/Diaphragm Breathing to have the best benefit in my practice with re-setting the vagus nerve. Perhaps it is because I actually practice it periodically during the day. I have also found it beneficial when I have tachycardia during the night.

For further direction, please visit my website: www.amgodin.com

EXERCISE

I know, I feel and hear you right now. Loud and clear. It's hard to exercise when you're chronically ill, but still . . . EXERCISE!

I know there are times you can barely function, let alone exercise. Believe me, I get it. I was there. But I'm not joking. So, let's not call it exercise, let's just call it movement.

Everyone has to start somewhere. If you are bedridden or couch bound, start small. Keep it simple. Here's an example: Today I will lift up my ankles and wiggle all my toes. I will lift my arms over my head and move my wrists and fingers.

Repeat the next day. Add in a few things as you progress, such as: Today I will sit up and put my feet over the side of the bed and raise my arms above my head.

Give yourself credit. Give gratitude for whatever you can do today. It is enough.

Please do not ever beat yourself up over not being able to accomplish what you did the day before or the week before. This, too, is not linear. Healing is not linear.

WALKING IS MOVEMENT.

STRETCHING IS MOVEMENT.

BREATH WORK IS MOVEMENT.

YOGA IS MOVEMENT. (IF YOU ARE ON THE MAT OR IN A CHAIR, IT IS STILL MOVEMENT.)

GARDENING IS MOVEMENT.

GOING UP AND DOWN YOUR STAIRS IS MOVEMENT.

Just move! The goal, the endgame, the touchdown is to heal and become fully functional. Do not set lofty goals that are unreasonable. Set safe, manageable, and realistic goals that you feel you can accomplish.

Whatever your energy level is that day, just choose to move. If you can eventually establish a routine that includes breath work, yoga or stretching, and walking, that's outstanding!

My own experience in this area is to not overdo it. Do not push your body too far or too fast or your body might push back . . . really hard. In the beginning, my body really struggled to identify what exactly was a stressor. Movement is good for you. But my body felt it was too much stress to do a regular movement routine and had zero reluctance in letting me know that it was too much. So, regular to me meant consistency. I did it every day. I committed to movement. Big or small, I committed to it.

It takes time, but you should eventually feel and see progression. You are not in competition with anyone but yourself. If you can do better than you have done before with movement, that is you raising the bar. Note: Give yourself the permission to rest. I mean fully rest, physically and mentally. Proper rest is healthy and necessary in healing.

I want to share a short story about movement. In the winter of 2020, I posted pictures of my husband and me out walking in minus-24-degree Celsius weather. It was a sunny and very cold day, and the ground was covered with newly fallen brilliant white snow. We were bundled up, but not too much because I like to keep my body cool. We took several pictures of the shadows of us holding hands together and of the beautiful landscapes. I posted the pictures, and most responses were wonderful. A few, however, were negative: You might fall. You might freeze. Minus twenty-four, are you crazy? Why would you do that?

Why? BECAUSE I CAN!

Because I can actually physically and mentally accomplish it. I vowed while I lay bedridden for way too long that movement was going to be a daily routine. That I was not going to waste one day without movement. Age has no bearing on movement, your health does. So, the WHY is because I bloody well am capable of doing it, so I bloody well will do it and with deep gratitude. I take absolutely nothing for granted!

To have access and download helpful lists, charts, and tools to assist with your health advocacy, please visit my website: www.amgodin.com

It is never too late in your life to feel and be your best. Don't let chronic illness make you feel as though your life is over or your most productive years are behind you. Here are some inspirational facts to prove that point:

An extensive study in *The New England Journal of Medicine* found that the most productive age in human life is between 60 and 70 years of age.

The second most productive stage of the human being is from 70 to 80 years of age.

The third most productive stage is from 50 to 60 years of age.

The average age of Nobel Prize winners is 62 years old.

The average age of presidents of prominent companies in the world is 63 years.

The average age of the pastors of the 100 largest churches in the US is 71.

The average age of a pope is 76 years.

It really does seem that the best years of your life are between 60 and 80 years.

The same study found that at age 60, you reach the top of your potential, and this continues into your 80s.

Lean in . . .

Transformation can be painful at times. Breaking habits and cycles is both painful and deeply rewarding. Letting go can sometimes be painful at first. The work that it takes to grow mentally and physically throughout the journey of healing is necessary because we are so worth it!

You are so worth it!

In early 2022, I turned 59. It's an amazing gratitude-filled gift, one some individuals never get to receive. So, buckle up, buttercup, as I am just reaching my stride of audacious and unapologetic awesomeness! I have the same positive thoughts about how you, too, can—with the right tools, knowledge, assistance, and attitude—step forward into healing.

Oh, it's been quite a journey. And I'm very proud of how far I've come, the growth I've accomplished, and the person I am now. From being bedridden and begging for someone to save me, I rose and found my footings, did a full pivot, and took the steps necessary to save myself.

You can do the same!

It feels like a gift to me to share, guide, and encourage you on your journey of healing.

CHAPTER 24

WHAT'S OLD IS NEW AGAIN

VIRAL PANDEMIC

December 31, 2019

(Wuhan Municipal Health Commission, China: Cluster of pneumonia cases reported in the area of Wuhan, Hubei Province. Eventually, a novel coronavirus is identified.)

With the growing concern over the vast number of cases, alarming rate of transmission, and severity, the World Health Organization confirms COVID-19 can be classified as a pandemic.

I reread the lines above and struggle to form my next sentence. Time has passed like a slow-moving train wreck. Hindsight is

20/20, and I think with this, like many other tragic events in life, when you know better, you do better. Humanity was not prepared for the crushing weight that COVID-19 would inflict upon us, mentally, physically, financially. Let alone the trail it would leave. Like a worldwide tornado, it swept in over a blue horizon, its enormity not fully registering until it was too late. It upended humanity with crushing, forbidding strength as we all paused and held our collective breath in a universal thread of hope.

I have chosen not to focus my thoughts on the "why" of it all. My purpose is mainly to express what it is like to live a life post-viral. I know how I felt post-viral before ever hearing about COVID-19 and still know how I feel today.

Some individuals have tragically lost their lives to COVID-19. My thoughts and sincere condolences to their loved ones. Others have recovered from COVID-19. Then there are those who are over the primary virus and are left with secondary syndromes, many of whom will have lingering physical and mental health issues because of the pandemic. They will feel just as invisible as the disease that took them down. Some will be left with post-viral syndromes that will also be just as invisible. They will feel many things on this part of the journey. All those emotions will come in waves like the largest of roller coasters with no one operating the controls. The cars slipping and sliding over the edge, screeching metal on metal as individuals hang on for their lives with no safety net and no harness as they try to catch their breath. Some gripping on with fingernails bitten to the quick as they embark on a steep and scary climb on their journey toward the long haul of living with chronic illness, and possibly despair.

I can't talk for others; I can only speak on behalf of myself and some others I know well who have been suffering with post-viral and other causes of chronic illness prior to COVID-19. We are the original "long haulers," before it was a label, before it was a hashtag. I don't say that out of pity, more out of experience in the "been there, done that, got the T-shirt" way. The experience of living with life after becoming chronically ill. The experience of dealing with the medical system, tests, medications, and treatments—or lack thereof. The experience of mentally, physically, and emotionally HEALING!

Honesty is the best policy . . . until honesty hurts, makes you think, makes it real, makes it painful. Well, here comes my brutally honest and honestly brutal truth. This pandemic journey is going to be the hardest, rockiest, and most painful mental, physical, and spiritual journey you have ever been on. I don't want it to sound all doom and gloom without hope. I do, however, feel it is crucially important to render a learning to the world we knew prior to the pandemic that life will not be the same after the pandemic. I feel you cannot go to hell and back without some degree of being burned. You cannot battle in a war and come out unscathed. As with any war, there will be wounds visible that fester and weep and that make us want to cover our eyes—wounds that we cannot unsee. Also, as with any war, there will be the invisible wounds that will fester, weep, and reopen, only to fester and weep yet again.

What I can say about a post-viral and past trauma. In the beginning of my illness, I felt so happy, so blessed to be alive. I was filled with so much gratitude that I survived. That I survived the initial illness and came out on the other side. What I didn't expect was that I wasn't going to be cured. Honestly, that isn't even the correct word, cured. I didn't expect that life wasn't going to be the same is more accurate. I really thought I'd be back to my old normal. In my naivety, I thought that once I had survived the initial onset, I would fully recover, utterly and completely, physically, emotionally, financially, spiritually. I did survive, but I wasn't the same. Not only did I survive, but I also miraculously moved forward into a new journey of healing and growth.

TWO STEPS FORWARD, ONE STEP BACK

As time progressed and reality set in for the majority of the world, the weeks turned into months. The months then turned into years, and here we are in a full-on pandemic that just keeps giving. I think it's quite normal to fear the unknown, the uncertainty of it all.

I have worked hard to heal. I've put in the time and have had success. And I have to say, the pandemic brought up old memories of the invisible viral disease that caused my chronic illness.

It brought back short blips in time that I had forgotten or tried to erase to ease my discomfort. It brought back a visual of the stages of grief, laid out in view for me to walk through to get full closure.

I remember one of my first days out of the house after being bedridden for almost a year. Sure, I had stretched my legs in the house. Having a back-split family home was a blessing and a curse, all in one. The multilevel house presented a challenge going up and down the stairs. It also gave the blessing of peace and quiet from the basement level to my bedroom on the top floor. Year one was mainly lived on the fourth level, with short trips to the kitchen. I had ventured out to our backyard in occasional short stints, and for the most part, those mini excursions had been successful, were peaceful, and brought solace. This particular day, however, was a big step compared to how I had been managing. I was so looking forward to the day of bonding with my soon-to-be daughter-in-law. I had convinced myself I could go on an outing and felt confident starting out. We planned on going to the local bookstore, chatting, and enjoying each other's company.

As soon as I got in the car, the smell seemed overpowering. I couldn't quite place it. Was it a "new car" smell? Was it an air freshener? Was it just an overly chemical plastic smell? It mattered not. I felt my senses being overwhelmed. I did my best to make chitchat, but brain fog was starting to ebb in. As we pulled into the vast parking lot at the mall in front of the bookstore, I felt relief wash over me, as I was hopeful the blast of fresh air when getting out of the car might slap back the brain fog and slap a fake smile on my face. It was my mask to wear in times of discomfort and is one I'm sure others will relate to.

The fresh air felt good as we walked briskly to the store. Once a haven for me with shelves lined with books and filled with the hustle and bustle of like-minded individuals walking aimlessly throughout aisles searching for their next great read, this time I felt the store's walls close in on me. The smells of the people, the foods, the synthetic world around me was too much. And the lights were much too bright. I mustered up all the cheerfulness I could to tell Betsy to go ahead and get what she was after, and we'd meet up in fifteen minutes.

I quickly scurried over to an open chair with my head reeling, brain fog swirling. I became agitated as the thoughts raced in my head. Don't they think of others when they bathe in perfume or cologne? Don't they think of others with their stench of second-hand smoke? Each minute I waited seemed to tick by like an hour. Yet everything else seemed to streak by as if going in fast-forward. I felt wasted as if I had been drugged. The room started to swirl as the noise level seemed to boom off my ear drums. I glanced over at the double pane of glass angled like a V. I could see a reflection of someone familiar sitting on the other side, and I leaned forward to get a better look at her. The older woman was relatively put together in her black outfit as she looked back. I noted the shock of surprise on her face as she drew her hand to her mouth. Tears rolled down my cheeks as clarity set in, and I realized I didn't recognize myself. My face was gaunt, my hair over-processed and long. Thoughts of self-pity were interrupted by Betsy. "Are you okay? Maybe we should go now."

She was right. I had convinced myself I should not be a party pooper on the day, so I had shamed myself into going. The day was planned in advance when I was feeling up to it, but I had learned that the syndrome had a mind of its own and was as unpredictable as a hornet's nest.

I barely made it home that day. I gave a brave smile and did my best to get up the five steps to my bedroom, where I collapsed on the floor, hungry for air. My voice hoarse and weak. I couldn't yell out for help. When I did open my mouth to utter words, they were barely audible, the words slurring together like a finger painting, messy and wanting of comprehension.

I'm screwed, I thought.

I struggled to not black out. My body jerked and twisted. My teeth chattered rhythmically out of control. It came and went in waves with the contractions of my muscles. My lower diaphragm was unable to give little assistance in breathing. I don't know how long I was sprawled out on the floor. I just know my eyes regained focus and the faraway echoes of noise within the house became recognizable. Did I hear Betsy in the kitchen one floor down? I could make it there, I told myself. Rolling to my left side, I rocked myself to a kneeling position and crawled across the carpet. My bare knees burned as the synthetic fibers etched fine lines as I made my way out of the bedroom. I called out, but my voice was weak, and I was still slurring. Exhausted, I leaned against the wall, trying to avoid the opening of the bathroom door. I wanted so badly just to lie there on the cool marble floor, to soothe my flushed face, to shut my eyes, and to silently say, "I give up. Do your worst. Take me away. I'm done."

Something deep inside me said, "No, not today."

I pushed myself off the wall, my hands gripping the top step. Partially falling, partially sliding, I fell down the stairs. Bump, bump, bump! I remember the fire department there. I remember the IV going in. I remember the EMS saying something about a silent seizure. I remember a face saying their name as my world washed into darkness. I awoke in the hospital, as I had the last half dozen times, to bright lights and noises. The face whose name I could not remember seemed to be advocating for me, his arms crossed, insisting they keep me in. His voice in a pitch that sounded slightly demanding, yet fearful and pleading all at the same time. "You need to keep her here. I've brought her in the last six times over as many months. She's dying. You need to figure out why."

He turned back to look at me and realized I was awake. He forced a smile and walked toward me and patted my hand with his gloved one. "You're going to be fine. They will take care of you." He leaned in and whispered, "Demand they keep you in. State you feel eminent doom." Then he was gone, one of the many superheroes in this world.

I was released a few hours later after my vitals abruptly returned to normal. The ER doctors chalked it up to anxiety, saying it was probably all in my head. They didn't explain the symptoms I had on arriving or how they disappeared as quickly as they appeared. Oh well, off you go, on to the next patient.

Yes, I was alive. I could imagine the choir of people voicing their opinions about how I should be grateful. How I should be thankful. How I should see the silver lining in it all. As far as I could tell, this was all part of the journey of living with an unknown invisible illness. I did feel some relief when I knew I was going to live, but in that moment of time, however, I also felt intense pain and hunger. I was weighing in at only eighty-five pounds and was on the verge of being tube fed. My immune system was in hyper-response mode to every piece of food I put into my mouth. I can now say that I know what it feels like to almost starve to death. People often say they're starving when they really mean they're just ready for their next meal. My stomach was concave; every rib was showing.

I stared back at the reflection in the mirror of my emancipated face. My once-sparkling blue eyes now reflected a dead sea. It was as if the life had been sucked out of me. I was a shell of myself. Yes, I was alive, but I was no longer among the living. I was housebound other than for doctor visits and hospital trips.

The journey of the long haul was taking its toll, and my thoughts wondered to the darkest of depths as I wished the illness would have taken me swiftly, painlessly, and fast, not eating away at me like a carnivore. In the beginning, living post-viral was as close to hell on earth as I could describe. I would not wish it on my worst of enemies.

NOTE TO SELF

Not everyone appreciates honesty. And the method you choose to deliver that honesty is just as important as the words. Not everyone is ready for or wants the honesty of that message. It's okay to not have all the answers on subjects you are not knowledgeable about. Sometimes it's better to just say, "I don't have the answer, but I know someone who will have the answer." Sometimes it is best just to say nothing, as not everything requires a response.

Opinions are your personal view. Assumptions are guesses of narrative and motive. Honesty involves your view from your perspective. Not everyone thinks like you, nor do they have the same perspective. When someone is in need, offer empathy, understanding, kindness, compassion, inspiration, motivation, and encouragement, and hold space for them. Provide to those what you wish was provided unconditionally to you.

TAKE A MOMENT FOR YOURSELF

Breathe, Pause, Reflect . . .

I think that, right there, is the best advice, the best level of honesty. My best opinion I can summon up is to simply breathe, pause, and reflect.

I haven't been here before in a world crisis, in a global pandemic.

I think everyone is trying to do their best.

Take time to reflect on your past to see if you can look back and find an unplanned pivot from which you have successfully moved forward.

Take time for yourself. Self-care is crucial. Your physical health is a number one priority. Your mental health is a number one priority.

This pivot will perhaps give you more than one opportunity to access what has been working for you in your life. What nurtures you, what priorities need changing.

CHAPTER 25

NEVER SAY NEVER

2020 AND BEYOND

By the spring of 2020, the world from my view was still deep in chaos as the pandemic raged on. I restricted the amount of time I was on social media, as well as the news I wanted to see and listen to. Please don't get me wrong; I was concerned. In fact, I was horrified with the devastation the entire planet was going through. But in that moment, I needed a bit of peace. I needed to see a funny post. I needed to read about a feel-good story going on in the world. I needed to spend time with family as we all adjusted to life.

Thankfully, our family remained healthy, although with careers in entertainment, real estate, education, and medicine, our sons, Jason, Joshua, Jordan and daughters-in-law Amy, Betsy, and Tea faced trying times on the work front. Our grandson has had the balance of being at home and in daycare. Our niece Laurel has a small business, which has seen several closures. "It is what it is" seems to be the common sentence I use. We all do the best we can. I try my best to be supportive, as I feel everyone has more stress in various forms to deal with than I do. I feel gratitude every day for what we do have.

I start each new day with stretching, morning meditation, and breath work. I have a cup of organic black coffee while I check emails and social media, then it's on to my yoga. I have established a new routine since we moved to the lake house. I fill the rest of my day with other wonderful things that I never really had time to fit in when I worked full time and had kids and dogs and all the busyness that life entailed. My life now feels full. I often wonder how the hell I got everything done when I worked full time. Am I right?! I can't be the only one who thinks that.

Our kids think Jeff and I have all the time in the world to get things done, now that we're retired. But it's funny how there's always a new routine to fill up one's day. The priority of things on the list to do is very different, but there's still a list that quickly fills up.

I walk daily, paint once a week or more, and write as if my life depends on it. Sometimes I really feel my life does depend on it.

I am a deep thinker, and most times, I find the quiet of the lake house aids the process. The words just spill out onto the pages—all the thoughts, emotions, joy, fear, and anxiety I feel. Sometimes the tears get in the way, but for the most part, the words blend with the tears in their own unique alchemy; their chemistry transforms an elixir, one that would be at a loss for the other.

One morning I eased into the morning emails as my phone chimed. I didn't recognize the phone number and debated answering it, as it's probably a telemarketer. By the third ring, my gut leaned in, and I answered the call that would result in another pivot. The volunteer from the Yorkie rescue organization was on the line with news that there were two small Yorkies who needed to be homed together.

I guess you should never say never, especially when you're a dog lover.

"Please don't email me the picture," I said to her.

"Too late, it's already sent. It's probably already in your inbox. Let me know what you think. The contact details and everything are in the body of the email," she said before saying goodbye.

I told myself not to open the email. I tried. I really did . . . for about one minute. Okay, it was more like fifteen seconds, if that. I opened the email and there they were: two adorable little peas in a pod. Their sad little faces looking at me, just wanting to be loved. I showed Jeff and started to read him the details as he got up and walked right past me.

"Babe, are you listening to me? OMG! Look at their little faces.

They have to go to the same home, as they're inseparable. Shit, it's a six-hour drive one way to get them. But babe, we would only have to cover the cost of—" Jeff was standing in front of me with his hat on and his car keys in his hand.

"Let's go! Grab your purse, some of your food, and your meds. Call her right now and say we're on our way." His voice was filled with "hurry up and move your ass; the babies are waiting."

The long drive was a breeze, and we chatted happily all the way. The paperwork and pickup went smoothly. It was meant to be, so easy that we laughed as we drove back, giggling as we repeated the phrase, "Start the car! Start the car!" as if we got the deal of a century and needed to get away before they figured it out.

And just like that, two more Yorkies entered our life, bringing us love, joy, and lots of laughs. We renamed them Ruby and Alfie. They had been neglected and were more than ready to be nurtured and loved as they so deserved. We rescued them, but more so, they rescued us. They brought a double ray of sunshine into our lives in a bleak time during COVID.

If there is one thing I have learned, it's that you can either let heartache make you bitter and hard, or you can let the wonderful memories fill your heart to remind you of the joy possible. Choose love. Always choose to love again.

NOTE TO SELF

I knew my statement of "never again" wasn't going to hold. It wasn't even a wall built, more like a flag heeding my heart in that moment of feeling overwhelmed and devastated at losing Abby. In that pain, my mind wanted to reaffirm what it didn't want my heart to bear again.

My heart, however, had other plans for expansion, renewal, and the quest to feel the flooding of positive emotions. My brain now thanks my heart for its brave choice to let the love and "happy hormone" dopamine flow, knowing that eventually it will again feel the pain of heartache. But living in the moment, I live with purpose, joy, love, and laughter. Without remorse and filled with gratitude, I say to go where your heart goes and the rest of you will follow.

TAKE A MOMENT FOR YOURSELF

Breathe, Pause, Reflect . . .

Volunteering with, visiting, and adopting from a shelter, nonprofit, or rescue situation can be rewarding for all if the right animal fits your lifestyle.

If you are chronically ill, having a pet can be a huge benefit, but it can also be a huge amount of work. However, to reap the benefits of an animal connection doesn't always equate to adoption.

Before we brought the new fur babies into our family, I helped out at our local wildlife rescue and visited the animals there.

Have you ever made a similar statement of "never again"? Have you ever eaten your words by doing that "never again" act yet again?

I have found it's much easier to recant those words if they involve an animal because of the unconditional love involved. Studies have shown that having a pet can reduce anxiety, depression, loneliness, and the stress-related hormone of cortisol. Pets can increase your positive feelings and elevate your mood.

IN CLOSING

We are living in a post-viral era. The sooner we, as in humanity, acknowledge the new world we're living in, the better off we will all be. When I indicate post-viral, I am referring to the aftermath of chronic illness that it leaves in its trail. I am not just referring to COVID-19 long haulers, I am including the countless number of individuals living with a chronic illness from an unknown virus. They are also long haulers.

Articles are being released at a rapid rate in correlation to COVID-19 long haulers, their actual underlying syndromes being autonomic nervous system dysfunction, such as dysautonomia. Some will have additional syndromes and disorders that also overlap with many other known disorders, such as myalgic encephalomyelitis/chronic fatigue syndrome (ME/CFS) and mast cell activation disorders.

In most instances, they are and remain like the virus—invisible to the naked eye.

The commonality for most is the immune system, vagus nerve, pathways, and possible gut microbiome. Studies are now showing the overlap of autoimmune diseases and the possible ability to promote a reset via stimulation to the vagus nerve.

According to the World Health Organization (WHO), at the time of writing, the number of individuals who had undiagnosed syndromes (pre-COVID-19) was estimated to be over 70 million. And according to WHO, chronic disease is estimated to rise substantially post-COVID-19 (whenever we actually reach the end of the pandemic). The strain on our medical systems, society, economy, and family structures will be dramatic indeed.

Some of those invisible diseases are chronic fatigue syndrome, mast cell activation syndrome, dysautonomia, post-infection disease syndrome, hyperimmune response syndrome, inflammatory response syndrome, and numerous other autoimmune diseases.

The post-viral health crisis started long before the pandemic. COVID-19 long haulers, however, have brought it front and center.

My goal in writing this book has been and always will be to give a voice to those not heard. To give hope to those who feel lost. To give understanding to those misunderstood. To allow the invisible to feel seen. And to raise awareness for the need of help and management, and to show that healing can be accomplished. My goal is to assist those who need a starting point and give a direction forward to healing.

As the fallout of COVID-19 continues, the numbers of long haulers continue to rise. Like all numbers in a health crisis, the full extent may not be known until the dust settles, and even then, it will take years to sort out the number of individuals affected by long-term health issues related to COVID-19.

It is encouraging, however, that more and more advocacy groups are emerging and support groups are popping up. In one breath, I am happy to see a recognition for those who feel invisible, and in another, I am so saddened to see that the need is there and that it's so high.

It is my utmost fear that people will fall through the cracks. And unfortunately, there are so many cracks to fall through as you battle your way through the long-term effects of living with chronic disease. People slip through the cracks medically, mentally, financially, and socially.

I have read many articles about how COVID long haulers are experiencing a lot of the same symptoms that other chronically ill (the original long haulers) have gone through due to a viral exposure. There are no markers in their test results. They go from doctor to doctor to doctor, looking for answers, looking for assistance, looking for a cure. Mainly, they are looking to feel "normal" again. They have lost so much of themselves that they don't know what it's like to now feel normal, let alone healthy. I say "they," but it should be a "we" in acknowledgment to those, myself included, who came before the long haulers of COVID-19. I give a solid nod of acknowledgment to those who came before, who have already walked that path, and who still walk the path.

Understanding what it is to be a long hauler is complex. It's easier to break down the illness into segments so that it can be better understood by both laymen and medical professionals.

We first have the primary illness. For this example, I'll use COVID-19-viral. An individual contracts the primary illness, then recovers, but they are left with ongoing symptoms that seem somewhat unrelated to COVID-19 symptoms overall. In some regards, those who have suffered through the primary virus have the "why" to their secondary disorders and symptoms that linger or evolve.

The unrelated symptoms, in actuality, are secondary disorders. It's like COVID-19 started a domino effect and the cascade has now opened up a plethora of new symptoms that are so vast and distinct that it's mind boggling. In most cases, individuals will end up with more than one "secondary" disorder to deal with. Those secondaries seem to fall into two categories: 1) stemming from autonomic nerve dysfunction and dysautonomia, and 2) hyperimmune response/hyper-inflammatory response including respiratory.

It's horrible to live with the invisible. People sometimes cannot perceive what they cannot see, even if they're members of the medical community. People's perceptions are based on their own experiences as well. If a disease or illness or long-term ramifications cannot be seen, some believe it does not exist. To all those COVID-19 long haulers, I am here to tell you, that's bullshit. It is not all in your head. It's real! It's tangible! It's horrific! It's unrelenting!

I must have gone through more than forty doctors and hundreds of tests—and nothing. Then I finally found a doctor who said, "Aha." Who ran specific testing to confirm my diagnosis. There isn't a gold seal test per se that can be used to measure what is going on for every disorder. Eventually, we could see testing that makes invisible diseases easier to diagnose, that shows antibodies to confirm, but not yet.

Dysautonomia itself is a beast. I describe my own as such. In the beginning, it was endless. In the beginning, when I spoke about it, I was terrified to poke the beast because once it awakens, I am taken down physically and mentally for weeks on end. When it flares, it attacks. And it doesn't take much to make it flare. I poignantly use the word "flare" because you will get to the point where you almost feel normal. Then the sleeping beast gets poked, and it awakens to remind you that it's still there. After the initial onset, mine has always functioned like an autoimmune disease where it has triggers and will flare up. If it walks like a duck and quacks like a duck, it is usually a duck. In my case, it's autonomic nerve dysfunction, and it's directly correlated with the immune system and possibly pathways. My protocol has diminished the flares substantially and durations of time for recovery.

February 24, 2021, was a somewhat historic day for Americans. Dr. Anthony S. Fauci, an American physician-scientist and immunologist serving as the director of National Institute of Allergy and Infectious Diseases since 1984 and Chief Medical Adviser to the past president and current President Joe Biden, made a formal announcement about a new syndrome. I needed to stop and gather my thoughts. I needed to pause.

Why?

The anger washed over me like rough seas, slapping my face. My cheeks became flushed, and I was intensely agitated. *USA Today* quoted Dr. Fauci as saying those "COVID-19 long haulers" will be known as the New Syndrome Post-Acute Sequelae of SARS-CoV-2 (PACE) to legitimize the suffering population. I have intense mixed feelings about that recent announcement. It's as if I can hear the roar of the mass number of people who feel heard, feel validated. Oh, trust me, I've been there. My emotions waver on elation for the COVID-19 long haul sufferers and devastation for all those who suffered from the same syndrome prior, without any recognition. The vast number of the worldwide population who have dysautonomia is estimated to be more than 70 million. The vast number of the worldwide population who suffer with mast cell and hyperimmune response is estimated to be more than 80 million. The vast number of the worldwide population who have fibromyalgia and chronic fatigue syndrome is estimated to be 120 million. The vast number of them had all these syndromes prior to COVID-19.

Do I think Dr. Fauci and his team did their due diligence? You would have to ask them. Are these syndromes isolated to just COVID-19 long haulers? Not at all—100 percent NO! Labeling it specifically to SARS-CV-2 is validating for some and defeating for others, who now may feel like their suffering is less important or legitimate. Was due diligence done to investigate with top experts around the world in all areas of the syndromes to name the combined syndromes a more generic or inclusive name? That's another question for Dr. Fauci and his team.

I have zero issues with them identifying why someone may have this syndrome. I do, however, have a huge concern that some in the medical community may be off target when looking at the underlying conditions, conditions that are not isolated to COVID-19 long haulers. These are conditions that have been around for quite a long time, some of which have treatments and medications and full-on community support and international groups. I foresee, unfortunately, a significant number of patients falling through the cracks and not getting treatment or a proper diagnosis for the secondary syndromes if it's connected to COVID-19. I can honestly hear the gaslighting now.

I am hopeful yet also apprehensive whether this labeling will restrict prior patients to the same level of care, treatment, management, or legitimization. Will it restrict patients in the future who did not get a COVID-19 test or possibly only had mild COVID-19 symptoms if they later develop secondary syndromes? How will those be treated if they don't fit nicely into the gold standard of the "why" and "where" of medicine? My heart breaks for anyone who will have to go through the frustration of not receiving the correct medical advice, medications, treatment, and support they so deserve.

I wish the medical community would instead focus more on the symptoms present rather than whether they fit into the slot of why this syndrome presents in the first place. Again, these syndromes and symptoms are not new to this world. I am not a doctor and do not give medical advice, but I can share my experiences of what it had been like to be a long hauler since 2012. I have the majority of the syndromes that most long haul COVID-19 sufferers have. I have dredged through the sludge. I have bankers' boxes filled with medical files, reports, research, and testing that ranges from the basic to the obscure.

I was a wealth adviser for the private division of a major Canadian bank. It's safe to say, I am a numbers person. I am logical, clinical, and detail oriented. I like to dot my i's and cross my t's. I am a puzzle solver and a pattern seeker. I also have a large creative streak that allows me to think outside the box. I like to look at the bigger picture. When tackling an issue, I want to get right down to the underlying problem. Keeping that in mind, I dissected my own syndromes and examined my health puzzle.

Currently, it has been stated that the estimation of long haulers is at 40 percent or greater, and of those, the majority, if not all, have the following:

Various medical articles state Post-Acute Sequelae of Coronavirus Disease 19 (Long Haul) show multi-systemic involvement. They also show confirmed secondary diagnoses heavily weighted in the following syndrome/diseases:

DYSAUTONOMIA

AUTOIMMUNE DISEASE

MAST CELL ACTIVATION / HYPERIMMUNE RESPONSE / HYPER-INFLAMMATORY RESPONSE

MYALGIC ENCEPHALOMYELITIS / CHRONIC FATIGUE SYNDROME

SMALL FIBER NEUROPATHY

FIBROMYALGIA

It's easy to see that there is, in fact, an overlap of symptoms, some commonalities.

In layman's terms, it seems the body's signaling or messaging systems have gone haywire. Inflammation is another commonality.

For my own research, I looked at those commonalities and looked for the thread as to why and where they could stem. After an exhausted search over years, I came to understand that my first inclination or gut instinct was sharper than I realized. I insisted that the severe GI issues that had continued to compound were making my overall syndromes worse. Why? The more I read, the more I realized that science was making groundbreaking traction in the connection between the immune system and the gut.

It was like an aha moment for me. I was hopeful, excited, and went on a rampage to fix my gut. Sounds simple, doesn't it? A few probiotics and clean eating and I would be back to normal. But it wasn't that easy. I crashed and burned and was left feeling defeated, just like I had with many other quick fixes.

The question became evident to me. How do you fix something when you can't get past the gatekeeper, which for me meant the immune system or the pathways/receptors in the gut to the immune system?

Why was the gatekeeper so confused about its purpose? In essence, I no longer cared about why the syndromes happened. I cared more about moving forward, where I was now, and what steps I had to take to have a better quality of life.

The question of why the gatekeeper acted a certain way changed to one of wondering where it was wounded or damaged.

This questioning brought me to my most profound link, connection, road map. What connects all the syndromes like an intricate human road map? What filters, instructs, and facilitates those directions? What crosses all aspects of the immune system, autonomic system, nerves, and messaging? Our first answer is naturally the brain. The second answer is the vagus nerve / pathways / receptors and it was my first directive of where the wounding or damage could possibly be.

So, here we all are . . . long hauling away. What are you going to do about it? You are possibly at a fork in the road. Frankly, you can't go back. You have choices, options. Do you turn left, or do you turn right? Honestly, I wish someone back in 2013 had told me to just turn, pivot, make a move, but don't stand still. Don't freeze. Whatever you do, don't remain stuck. Please pivot, shift focus. Step forward in whatever direction you must. Don't hold onto the preconceived notions of what you were prior to COVID-19.

This is where you are now, and this is what you are going to do about it.

It's time to pivot. It's time to make the pivot forward to healing!

Perception can only be truly conceived through living at the same level of existence and despair. All our journeys are different and as unique as we are. We do, however, have common threads. As a whole, humanity has the ability to reach a level of understanding that can bring kindness, compassion, and empathy.

To those who are long haulers, we have the depth of perception of one another's journey that has a way of getting it because of our "got it" attitude.

I am brutally honest and chronic illness has been honestly brutal. My writing brings that raw, unfiltered edge into the light without holding back, without shame.

I want more than anything to bring hope and understanding to many, but I'm content if it just reaches one, so they can realize they are not alone. Perhaps I am being modest here. I want to scream from the rooftops to reach the masses: "Do not lie quietly and accept that this is as good as it will get. Rise up! And if you can't, then lean the hell in, lean on, as there are more warriors like me who can and will support you. Speak up, speak out, speak even if your voice trembles. Take up space, then take up some more damn space. Hold space for others and gather a group that holds space for you. Keep yourself, your heart, and your mind open, remembering that being on a journey is an evolving process. Change happens—embrace it!"

It is not in your head. I want you to feel heard!

I want to encourage you to feel motivated to be the strongest, most driven badass health advocates you can be, so you can quest onward to a better quality of life. Each day, I hope you rise to realize that there is no competition with others. Furthermore, you are not in competition with your old self. You are enough!

Keep yourself open to exploring all different aspects of health and healing. Have a willingness to uncover the root, emotionally and medically. Have a willingness to expand your healing through exploring what mainstream does not provide, such as psychosomatic healing and regulation. My own journey with lessons on personal boundaries and self-advocacy highlighted is not only okay, but also necessary to sometimes draw a line in the sand with friends, family, the medical community, and society. Boundaries are self-care, and healing needs self-care.

Honor yourself. Honor your healing journey to trust your gut, to trust your instincts. Listen to your body and take in the message that it sends you. Understanding how emotions are deeply connected to our physical body and healing happens from the inside out.

I hope I have conveyed the essence of my journey, the physical, emotional, and mental struggle it brought. The depth of losses in life, including the devastating loss of oneself and all the grief that that entailed. Grief is a fact of life, though the perception by the majority is a visual or absence of a person or pet who has passed. Grief for the loss of oneself is much like the physical illness, invisible to others. Grief comes in many, many forms. It has no shelf life, no expiry date. The journey of grief is just a journey of its own that is as unique as the person is. My hope is that I have given some insight to the depths and also to the ways in which others, family, and friends can assist, not by solving, not by diminishing, but by empathy, compassion, understanding, and validation. I can't talk for others in how they compare the various emotions and feelings that come with grief, but I can say from my own experience that losing oneself has been the hardest grief journey I have ever walked. When others do not equate chronic illness to losing one's self, which can cause immense grief, the journey is made even more painful by individuals making your life much more difficult, more emotionally, physically, and mentally challenging.

Boundaries are there for you. They are not there as a punishment or a grudge. They are there because some individuals have toxic traits and behavior in trauma response that isn't conducive to your healing. They are placed as a safeguard to help protect the healing process and to live your life with healthy mutual relationships. The journey can be a painful, lonely one. Having a healthy support team is not only highly recommended, but it is highly beneficial in many ways. Let go of what does not nurture and help heal you.

We are in this together. You are not alone.

To all those women out there in the world, I hope you felt my words and emotions as they poured out onto the pages and that you now feel even more motivated to tap into your inner warrior in all areas of your life. Tap into your tenacity and claim your opportunities in life. Unsubscribe from society and finally live your own life. Honor the seasons of your life for what they are.

I intrinsically wanted to touch on the wound in the community of sisterhood. It's there; we all know it's there. Acknowledgment is half the battle. Imagine if each one of the women in the world said to themselves, *What am I going to do today that has a positive impact on myself and how can I transfer that positivity to other woman?* Lift others up. More specifically, lift other women up! Helen Reddy's 1971 "I Am Woman" was an anthem to motivate a united front of sisterhood. Perhaps we should collectively listen to the lyrics again. Let's judge less and clap more. Let's lift up, inspire, and motivate. Let's show empathy, understanding, and compassion. Let's not build walls, let's set tables for an inclusive community of strong women who are always ready to welcome another!

My wish during this worldwide crisis is for fear to turn into an awakening, one that opens the hearts of mankind and allows in the essence of life. We are all human, all vulnerable. Money, a big house, a jet plane, and luxury trips will not save you. The reality is that our treasures in life are the oxygen we breathe, the food we eat, and the relationships we nurture. Create joyful memories!

Be safe!

Sincerely,

Anne Marie Godin, The Long Hauler

RESOURCES

Maya Angelou, *The Oprah Winfrey Show*, 1997 episode, Harpo Productions

E. Azabou, MD, and G. Bao, PhD., et al., "Vagus nerve stimulation: a potential adjunct therapy for COVID-19," *Frontiers in Medicine*, May 7, 2021, https://www.frontiersin.org/articles/10.3389/fmed.2021.625836/full

Jeffrey S. Bland, PhD, "The Long Haul of COVID-19 Recovery: Immune Rejuvenation versus Immune Support," *Intergrative Medicine: A Clinician's Journal*, https://www.ncbi.nlm.nih.gov/pmc/articles/PMC7819497/

Dan Brennan, MD, "What is Mast Cell Activation Syndrome?" published April 12, 2021, www.webmd.com/allergies/what-is-mast-cell-activation-syndrome

Melanie Dani, MD, et al. "Autonomic dysfunction in 'long COVID': rationale, physiology and management strategies," *Clinical Medicine*, Royal College of Physicians, January 2021, www.ncbi.nlm.nih.gov/pmc/articles/PMC7850225/

Glennon Doyle on Instagram: linktr.ee/glennondoyle (www.instagram.com/glennondoyle/)

Jackie Dunham, "Doctors warn of possible rise of debilitating nervous-system disorder in patients with long COVID-19," CTVNews.ca, October 7, 2021, www.ctvnews.ca/health/coronavirus/doctors-warn-of-possible-rise-of-debilitating-nervous-system-disorder-in-patients-with-long-COVID-19-19-1.5615322

Douglas Fox, "Can Zapping the Vagus Nerve Jump-Start Immunity?" *Scientific American*, May 4, 2017, www.scientificamerican.com/article/can-zapping-the-vagus-nerve-jump-start-immunity/

Roger Gabriel, "How to Use Sound to Heal Yourself," January 15, 2015, https://chopra.com/articles/how-to-use-sound-to-heal-yourself

Robert Howland, MD, "Vagus Nerve Stimulation," The National Center for Biotechnology Information, published June, 2014, www.ncbi.nlm.nih.gov/

John Hopkins Medicine, Postural Orthostatic Tachycardia Syndrome (POTS); The Friend Who Keeps You Young, www.hopkinsmedicine.org/

M.J. Kenney and C.K. Ganta, "Autonomic Nervous System and Immune System Interactions," July 2014, www.ncbi.nlm.nih.gov/pmc/articles/PMC4374437

Dr. Elisabeth Kübler-Ross, *On Death and Dying: What the Dying Have to Teach Doctors, Nurses, Clergy and Their Own Families (50th anniversary)*, 2014, Scribner

Caroline Leaf, PhD, "How to Use the Neurocycle to Break Cycles, Heal Generational Trauma & End Toxic Family Patterns + How the Neurocycle Influences Epigenetics & Changes Genes," drleaf.com, posted March 4, 2021.

National Institute of Neurological Disorders and Stroke, Dysautonomia Information Page, www.ninds.nih.gov/

Shawn Radcliffe, PhD, "Long COVID Linked to Unbalanced Gut microbiome: What to know now," published January 27, 2022, www.healthline.com/health-news/long-covid-linked-to-unbalanced-gut-microbiome-what-to-know-now

Pratik Sinha, PhD; Michael A. Matthay, MD; Carolyn S. Calfee, MD, "Is a 'Cytokine Storm' Relevant to COVID-19?" June 30, 2020, *JAMA Internal Medicine*, https://jamanetwork.com/journals/jamainternalmedicine/fullarticle/2767939

Andrea Stofkova, PhD, and Masaaki Murakami, PhD, "Neural activity regulates autoimmune diseases through the gateway reflex," published August 20, 2019, https://bioelecmed.biomedcentral.com/articles/10.1186/s42234-019-0030-2

Peter Novak, MD, PhD, et al., "Multisystem Involvement in Post-Acute Sequelae of Coronavirus Disease 19," *Annals of Neurology: An Official Journal of the American Neurological Association and the Child Neurology Society*, published December 24, 2021, https://doi.org/10.1002/ana.26286

The British Medical Journal, "Gut microbiota dynamics in a prospective cohort of patients with post-acute COVID-19 syndrome," bmj.com

The New England Journal of Medicine, www.nejm.org/ 70.389, 2018

Zarlakhta Zamani, MD, and Utsav Parekh, MD, "Vanishing Twin Syndrome," The National Center for Biotechnology Information, updated July 21, 2021, www.ncbi.nlm.nih.gov/books/NBK563220/

YGTMedia Co. is a blended boutique publishing house for mission-driven humans. We help seasoned and emerging authors "birth their brain babies" through a supportive and collaborative approach. Specializing in narrative nonfiction and adult and children's empowerment books, we believe that words can change the world, and we intend to do so one book at a time.

ygtmedia.co/publishing

@ygtmedia.company

@ygtmedia.co

www.ingramcontent.com/pod-product-compliance
Lightning Source LLC
Chambersburg PA
CBHW070053030426
42335CB00016B/1871
9781989716601